Rapid changes are taking place in the practice of psychiatry and nowhere is this more pronounced than in its community aspects. Much has changed and this sometimes appears to have done so without adequate forethought or research although there is already a considerable body of knowledge that underscores recent developments. In this book prominent researchers in this expanding subject debate the implications of recent knowledge derived from a variety of sources and look ahead at impending developments that will need further research inquiry. The chapters are wide in scope and topical in content and the discussions after each are frank and informative. This book will be of help to all those involved in the organisation of psychiatric care.

COMMUNITY PSYCHIATRY IN ACTION:
ANALYSIS AND PROSPECTS

COMMUNITY PSYCHIATRY IN ACTION: ANALYSIS AND PROSPECTS

Edited by

PETER TYRER

Professor of Community Psychiatry
Academic Unit of Psychiatry
St Charles' Hospital, London, UK

and

FRANCIS CREED

Professor of Community Psychiatry
Rawnsley Building
Manchester Royal Infirmary
Manchester, UK

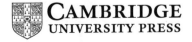

CAMBRIDGE
UNIVERSITY PRESS

Published by the Press Syndicate of the University of Cambridge
The Pitt Building, Trumpington Street, Cambridge CB2 1RP
40 West 20th Street, New York, NY 10011–4211, USA
10 Stamford Road, Oakleigh, Melbourne 3166, Australia

First published 1995

Printed in Great Britain at the University Press, Cambridge

A catalogue record for this book is available from the British Library

Library of Congress cataloguing in publication data

Community psychiatry in action : analysis and prospects / edited by
Peter Tyrer and Francis Creed.
p.   cm.
Includes index.
ISBN 0 521 47427 2 (hc)
1. Community mental health services.   2. Community psychiatry.
3. Community mental health services – England.   4. Community
psychiatry – England.   I. Tyrer, Peter J.   II. Creed, Francis.
[DNLM: 1. Community Mental Health Services.   WM 30 C733426 1995]
RC45.5.C61746   1995
362.2′2 – dc20
DNLM/DLC
for Library of Congress   94–35007 CIP

ISBN 0 521 474272 hardback

EBF

Contents

Contributors

Dr Tom Burns
St George's Hospital Medical School, Jenner Wing, Cranmer Terrace, Tooting, London SW17 0RE, UK

Professor Francis Creed
Rawnsley Building, Manchester Royal Infirmary, Oxford Road, Manchester M13 9WL, UK

Dr Christine Dean
Centre for Mental Health Services, King's College, Campden Hill Road, London W8 7AH, UK

Dr Brian Ferguson
Consultant Psychiatrist, Stonebridge Centre, Cardiff Street, Carlton Road, Notttingham NG3 2FH, UK

Dr Frank Holloway
St Giles' Psychiatric Day Hospital, St Giles' Road, Camberwell, London SE5 7RN, UK

Professor Martin Knapp
Personal Social Services Research Unit, The University, Canterbury, Kent CT2 7NZ, UK

Professor Isaac Marks
Institute of Psychiatry, De Crespigny Park, Denmark Hill, London SE5 8AF, UK

Professor Peter Tyrer
Academic Unit of Psychiatry, St Charles' Hospital, London W10 6DZ, UK

Dr Til Wykes
Clinical Psychologist, Institute of Psychiatry, De Crespigny Park, Denmark Hill, London SE5 8AF, UK

1

Essential issues in community psychiatry
PETER TYRER

Introduction

Community psychiatry is a portmanteau couplet that can mean many different things. To some it merely seems to imply 'extra-mural' psychiatry (i.e. any mental health care that goes on outside the walls of hospitals), to others it represents a specific form of care that involves particular skills and procedures and to others still it appears to be a form of policy to close outdated hospitals. This book focuses on the essential elements of research in community psychiatry and, as an initial task in research is to define exactly what is being measured, we need to define our terms before proceeding to research inquiry. This chapter is concerned with four main issues; the components of community psychiatry, their effectiveness, the development of the results of research into clinical practice and the proper focus of research in the subject.

What are the essential components of community psychiatry?

Community psychiatry is at different times a government policy, a planning strategy and a method of delivering psychiatric care. The first two of these are not open to research in the same way as the third and sometimes seem to be ignored or derided by research workers as they are not based on hard data. They are, however, fundamental in community psychiatry because they emphasise the importance of society in implementing the care of the mentally ill. Society decided in the early and middle years of the nineteenth century that patients with significant mental illness should be cared for in asylums where they should be protected from others in society. Exceptions could be construed as either benevolent or punitive depending on one's point of view but they enjoyed the consensus of opinion at the time and are regarded as advances.

1

In the early years of this century the policy was questioned in various countries but the mental hospital population continued to grow in most Western countries until the 1940s and 1950s. At that time society became suddenly concerned about the negative influences of large institutions, including mental hospitals (Goffman, 1961) with repeated complaints about the negative therapeutic influences of such institutions and the more enlightened views of society which helped to de-stigmatise the mentally ill, the process of de-institutionalisation and the growth of community psychiatry began. The Government White Paper, *Better Services for the Mentally Ill* (1975) summarised this approach and the ensuing 20 years have maintained it in almost identical form. In summary, the approach states that wherever possible patients should be treated in the settings that are most appropriate for the optimal care of their disorder and this could include their own homes, the surgeries of general practitioners, hospital outpatients clinics, day hospitals and various forms of inpatient care.

Effectiveness

A core component of research into treatments in medicine is the assessment of benefits and risks and the first of these can be summarised under the heading of efficacy. It is now appreciated worldwide that the best way of assessing the efficacy of a treatment is through the procedure known as the randomised controlled trial. This approach, first formalised by Austin Bradford Hill over half a century ago, attempts to control for all elements of treatment apart from the specific treatments under investigation and, when combined with accurate and reliable measurements of outcome, allows conclusions to be made about the value of the treatment separated from all other factors.

Research into the efficacy of services is more difficult because the isolation of the critical elements is often impossible to achieve. It can also be argued that it is the combination of elements rather than one or two individual ones that makes a good service, and that to isolate them is an artificial exercise. The standard research design for assessing efficacy of services is still, nevertheless, the randomised controlled trial, despite its many limitations. This issue is responsible for much of the debate in the last chapter of this book. It is an important debate that should help in working out the best way of evaluating these services in the future.

The Department of Health, who co-sponsored the symposium which forms the basis of this book, are also in the midst of health service reforms that affect many aspects of psychiatric care. Among these is the separation of 'purchasers' (those who represent the population who have needs for mental health services) and 'providers' (the services available to meet these needs). The purchasers, if they are to perform their task effectively, need to know whether the providers are adequately resourced and whether their services are delivered in the right way. In short, they need to measure efficacy and its more nebulous cousin, quality. They are desperately seeking measures that enable different services to be compared for effectiveness and models that can be used to predict the effects of service change.

Research organisations at all levels are involved in this search and while at present the comparative evidence is at a relatively primitive level (e.g. whether community-based care is superior to hospital-based care for a specific group of patients) it is moving forward fast. Efficacy also needs to be assessed at several levels; the relief of mental distress, the ability to function well in society, the quality of life achieved, the cost of the service, satisfaction of referrers, patients and their relatives and the degree of protection from relapse. This is clearly not just the specific goal of effective treatments in community psychiatry but whereas earlier studies have been concerned with relatively selected populations (e.g. patients with schizophrenia who are regular clinic attenders), community psychiatry is a subject that covers whole populations. A service may be excellent in its management of 40% of the sufferers from a certain mental illness but its value will be greatly reduced if it fails to reach the 60% who still need care but who never reach the service.

What should be the focus of research in community psychiatry?

It is an unfortunate fact that research tends to focus on what can be easily researched rather than what is most important. There is also a danger when standard research strategies do not seem to be possible that the substitute of a mere description of the service or a development is sufficient to enthuse others. Unfortunately, as there are probably as many ways of delivering community psychiatric services as there are individuals within the service this approach is not likely to prove of general value. The tremendous variation that exists between types of service, nevertheless emphasises the need for flexibility in implementing any model of care.

There has been much attention in recent years to the organisation of community psychiatric care. This when stimulated particularly by the development of case management in the USA has a form of delivery care. There are many models of case management, including ones in which the whole team acts as a case manager and individual patient, right down to a loose structure in which administrative responsibility is held by one individual or group but care is given by others.

In the UK care management and care programming now have specific meanings (Department of Health, 1990). Care programming is intended to be given to all those referred to the specialist mental health services and, despite its name, is meant to reinforce existing good practice rather than provide an alternative structure for care. Care management is specifically identified for those with severe and enduring mental illness who have many needs that require careful assessment (e.g. dementia treated at home, people with schizophrenia who are unable to live independently even when treated adequately). Social services and other organisations independent of the health (provider) sector are often the main assessors of such needs and have the resources to realise them but to varying degrees they involve other professionals in making their assessments. A detailed care plan is created as a consequence of this assessment and is subsequently monitored and reviewed at regular intervals.

Unfortunately the wording of these approaches is somewhat confusing, not least because 'case management' was the term first used to describe the careful monitoring and after-care of psychiatric patients discharged from hospital. The fundamental component of good case management is the need for the service to follow the patient wherever he or she goes in the psychiatric or social system. The success of this approach was first conclusively demonstrated by Stein & Test (1980) in a pioneering study in Madison, Wisconsin. They demonstrated that, when patients presenting for admission were allocated to hospital care or intensive home-based treatment by community psychiatric teams, the number of admissions and bed occupancy were much less in the community-treated patients at follow-up, patient and relative satisfaction were greater and social functioning better in the community treated sample. The model of this research was replicated again in the Daily Living Project described in Chapter 2 of this book. Similar results were found by Hoult and his colleagues (Hoult & Reynolds, 1985; Hoult, 1986) in Australia. Both groups of workers found that community care given in this way was somewhat cheaper than standard care because hospital costs were reduced greatly.

These findings are relatively easy to replicate if resources are available and, to a large extent, have been confirmed in the studies described in this book. There are several other elements, however, that could be focused on now in research studies.

Costs are a highly relevant issue. All health service systems are constrained by financial resources and if two models of care are roughly identical in efficacy then the cheaper one will inevitably attract more attention and be preferred in most psychiatric services. Costs are not necessarily easy to measure and the discipline of health economics has grown rapidly in the past few years as the importance of the subject has received proper attention. The subject of costs therefore appears repeatedly throughout the pages of this book and is addressed in detail in Chapter 10. Recording the exact costs involved in treating the patient is a much more difficult subject than it first appears but the identification of those groups of patients that cost the most money to the psychiatric services is a necessary prerequisite of good service management.

The skills and handicaps involved in community psychiatric work also are deserving of research attention. They are difficult to research adequately and are rarely the subject of randomised controlled trials but they can often make the difference between a successful community psychiatric service and one that is abandoned as a hopeless form of care.

We also need to know much more about the handicaps and disadvantages of working in community psychiatric teams. It is all very well demonstrating that a programme of treatment is successful in a research setting, where a range of motivations is present apart from the inherent wish to provide a good service, and quite another thing to extend this to normal everyday practice. There is much talk of burn-out in community psychiatric staff. Exactly what this means is difficult to tell but certainly many staff seem to opt for a quieter life in more settled surroundings after they have been involved in some of the programmes that have been described in the research literature. At the same time many programmes are continuing independent of research activity; perhaps the Madison experiment is the best known and this continues to operate in the same general mode as when it was first described nearly 15 years ago. The evidence seems to be that long-term community psychiatric care is both good for patients and satisfying for community teams but we need much more evidence to be certain of this and it would be a great help if we knew exactly what negative factors made some community psychiatric teams fail, sometimes very shortly after they had been set up. This is addressed in Chapter 9 by Wykes in discussing the 'toxicity' of community care. Just in the same way that all treatments have unwanted effects, all types of psychiatric service can have unwanted effects and we need to have these brought out into the open so that they can be dealth with positively.

There is also the very important question of morale to take into account. There are great difficulties in measuring morale and there are many factors that impinge on its presence but this is a critical factor that may determine the success or failure of a community team, or indeed any other psychiatric service. A great deal seems to depend on what is described in business circles as 'corporate identity'. If the team feels it has a common purpose and a common philosophy it is able to overcome an immense number of potential handicaps, whereas if it is fragmented and faction-ridden it will disintegrate at the first sign of external conflict.

To achieve a common purpose it would be helpful to have common training for all community teams. At present, at least in the UK, training is entirely led by individual disciplines within mental health. The training received by each discipline is different and the combination of beliefs and attitudes inculcated is such that when these disciplines are put together later and asked to work in a community team a potentially explosive mixture is produced. If social workers and occupational therapists are taught that diagnosis is a dangerous practice that 'labels' patients and dehumanises them, they are not likely to collaborate well with other staff, mainly psychiatrists, who are taught from the beginning of their training that diagnosis is an essential element of assessment. Similarly, psychologists taught in behavioural and cognitive therapies find it equally difficult to collaborate with staff trained in psychodynamic methods who regard behavioural theory as reductionistic and inappropriate for most patients' needs. When one adds the mix of the extremes of psychiatry between those of 'organic' adherence who regard all psychiatric disturbance as biologically determined to those who regard every psychiatric problem as a unique psychodynamic event that cannot be classified further, it is easy to see how conflict can become the norm when these team members sit down together to discuss the problems of their patients.

How do we develop research advances?

In recent years it has become obvious that many apparent research advances are not being implemented in practice. This applies across the field of medicine and has led to a re-examination of priorities. The Department of Health has set up a Research and Development section which is concerned both with the commissioning and implementation of research. The expectation is that when research advances are made in the R & D programme these can cascade downwards to everyday practice so that within a matter of 2–3 years they are implemented and are showing their effect on a national scale. There is now abundant evidence that major research advances are far too slow to be incorporated into ordinary practice and that far too often many more research studies are carried out than are really necessary to demonstrate that an advance has truly been made.

What is missing is the rapid transfer of the advance to clinical work. In psychiatry the academic component of the subject has sometimes been held in less regard than it could have been because so much of what goes on in psychiatric academia seems to lead to no improvement in clinical practice. This is perhaps unfair because the essential link between the research development and its implementation does not seem to be present. This is not so true of other areas of medicine. For example, the demonstration that cot deaths could be reduced significantly by ensuring that young babies lay on their sides or back rather than on their front has been immediately introduced into clinical practice (admittedly with the aid of an effective media campaign) and has led to a dramatic reduction in the incidence of cot deaths.

There is no such parallel in psychiatry and this also includes community psychiatry also. Advances which appear clear cut and easy to implement, such as the demonstration that by reducing high levels of expressed emotion relapse in schizophrenia is reduced significantly (Vaughn & Leff, 1973) have not been implemented satisfactorily into clinical practice. It is only now, after the publication of this original research, that clinical services are accepting the implications and training their staff, particularly community psychiatric nurses, accordingly.

One of the problems in implementing research is that it is often expensive. There is no point in developing a highly effective but extremely expensive new treatment of a condition that is extremely common unless one can predict with some confidence that the expense will reduce over time and become an alternative that will be available for most people in a National Health Service. If the new treatment involves many hours of training and skill development there are additional problems and this is accentuated if refresher courses or further training is necessary to maintain the skills of practitioners. In evaluating community psychiatric services there are particular difficulties that are not encountered when evaluating specific treatments. A service involves the package of ingredients that are difficult to separate from each other in the clinical sense, although they can be in strict research terms. A useful parallel is the evaluation of dietary habits. It is possible to identify each of the different ingredients in a three course meal and to carry out experiments about the negative and positive effects of each type of food. A great deal of information can be obtained from such studies, such as the demonstration that a diet high in saturated fats is likely to lead to a greater incidence of atheroma and heart disease, that high vegetable and fruit consumption reduces this risk and that foods containing sugar promote dental caries, but nutritionists have found it much more difficult to change dietary habits than might at first have been appreciated. There appear to be rituals and traditions bound up with eating that are difficult to change and the demonstration of long-term handicaps of particular foods do not seem to be regarded as too important by many members of the population. Of course, every so often there are some special dangers that are highlighted that do lead to changes in habits. The possible fatal interaction of rhubarb and spinach in those few people who mix these two foods or eat them consecutively, is a case in point.

So it is with developments in community psychiatric services. Which of the ingredients of home visiting, liaison with primary care, multi-disciplinary team function, the presence of a community team base or better liaison with hospital services constitutes the most important component of a good service and how many are redundant or of trivial importance? The secondary question such as the actors that ensure the durability of good community teams also need to be addressed.

These questions are often dismissed by pure scientists as part of the most minor form of operational research, although they are at least of equal importance to the more fundamental questions about whether a particular approach is 'effective' in the strict treatment sense.

Investigations of these issues often come under the heading of what is called 'action research'. This differs considerably from the randomised controlled trial. The latter can investigate the relative effects of 20 different variables in a service but the time and trouble taken in doing so is prohibitive. We have to examine a range of different functioning systems and use common measures to determine their efficacy, following which it is possible to get a reasonable notion of the features that facilitate good functioning and those which handicap it.

Once the ideal form of service is determined and the most reliable means of delivering it are found, we have a combination that can be repeated in many parts of the country. It is only at this stage that one can decide on what training and other facilities are needed so that similar teams can be set up in different areas. In the same way that the nutritionist will not get very far in training the dietary habits of the nation by issuing broad advice such as 'eat more brussel sprouts and broccoli', the planners of psychiatric services will have a similar negative response if they issue proclamations such as 'most psychiatric patients should be seen at home'. A blend of measures, with sufficient flexibility to account for the different geographical and social needs of populations, is necessary to effect useful change.

This book represents such a blend. It represents the deliberations and debates of a symposium that was held between most of the main researchers in UK community psychiatric care on the 4 March 1993 at the Royal College of Physicians in London. The presentations included accounts of research studies carried out in different parts of the country that included sufficient measurements to conclude with some confidence what accounted for the changes in each instance. To extend the nutritional metaphor, these contributions form the meat of the sandwich but they were garnished by critical accounts from other experts (there are few people more reformed and critical than fellow research workers) and accompanied by a wide ranging discussion of the possible ways forward for research in community psychiatry. This discussion is brought together in the final chapter in which many of the arguments and tensions involved in future work were aired and discussed constructively.

The result is a topical and honest reflection of the difficulties in research in an important and developing subject, which in some quarters is seen as being out of control and it is being driven by considerations other than clinical and research needs. We hope that the reader will agree that we have made a reasonable attempt to rein in the wild community horse and to train it sufficiently to become a useful servant for our psychiatric patients.

References

Department of Health (1990). *Caring for people: community care in the next decade and beyond*. CM849, HMSO, London.

Goffman E (1961). *Asylums*. Doubleday, New York.

Stein LJ, Test MA (1980). Alternative to mental hospital treatment. 1. Conceptual model treatment program and clinical evaluation. *Archives of General Psychiatry*, **37**: 392–7.

Hoult J (1986). Community care of the acutely mentally ill. *British Journal of Psychiatry*, **149**: 137–44.

Hoult J, Reynolds I (1985). Schizophrenia: a comparative trial of community oriented and hospital oriented psychiatric care. *Acta Psychiatrica Scandinavica*, **69**, 359–72

Vaughn CE, Leff JP (1973). The influence of family and social factors on the course of psychiatric illness: a comparison of schizophrenic and depressed outpatients. *British Journal of Psychiatry*, **93**, 129: 125–37.

2

Evaluation of community treatments for acute psychiatric illness

FRANCIS CREED

Overview of UK studies

Introduction

The growth of community treatment programmes for acute psychiatric illness has provoked considerable discussion in relation to both service development and research. On the one hand, the 'enthusiasts' for community treatments argue that this is the superior form of care and imply that every district should switch their resources from hospital to community treatment. On the other hand, critics argue that the superiority of community treatment has yet to be firmly established, either pointing out weaknesses in the research or insisting that any beneficial effects are probably marginal, related to the enthusiasm of the staff involved and that the real costs (e.g. possible increased suicide rate or 'burn-out' of staff) have yet to come to light. The argument tends to highlight the missionary zeal of the community enthusiasts and the defensiveness of the traditionalists rather than being based on sound scientific principles. The research findings to date are not sufficiently persuasive to end the argument.

The studies most widely quoted in favour of the community approach are those of Stein & Test (1980) and Hoult (1986); as these are outside the UK they can be criticised or supported with a degree of detachment. This is not so for the recent UK studies; the results of these local studies need to be examined firstly, to inform decisions about how UK community psychiatric services might be developed (including how they may contribute to 'Health of the Nation' targets) and secondly, to establish the next generation of research questions (Rosen, 1992; NIMH, 1991).

There have been five recently completed UK studies. In this brief review the results are compared to answer the following questions:

(1) Can a meta-analysis of the UK studies be performed?
(2) Is there evidence that such treatment programmes can be:
   (a) generalised to districts other than the site of the experimental programme?
   (b) sustained over a period of time: does the nature of the service change with time?

The studies to be considered are the following:

(1) Home based care for patients with severe mental illness (Muijen *et al.*). This will be referred to as the Daily Living Programme (DLP)
(2) Early intervention in psychiatric emergencies (Merson *et al.*, 1992). The Early Intervention Study (EIS)
(3) Home based service for acute psychiatric patients (Burns *et al.*, 1993). The St George's service.
(4) Day hospital for acute psychiatric illness (Creed *et al.*, 1991*a*). The Manchester day hospital study.
(5) Home treatment for acute psychiatric illness (Dean C & Gadd, 1990). This was not a random allocation study but is included as it is a potentially comparable programme to the others. It will be referred to as the Birmingham study.

Possibility of a meta-analysis

Performing a meta-analysis requires that the samples of patients included in each experimental programme are similar; the data presented below demonstrate that they are not. An alternative approach would be to identify subgroups, which are comparable, within different studies. This would be difficult without special further analyses.

The patients treated in the different programmes differ with respect to their selection, demographic features and severity of illness/diagnosis.

Selection of patients

The patients selected for the different experimental treatment programmes were as follows:

(A) DLP: serious mental illness requiring immediate hospital admission.
(B) EIS: psychiatric emergencies presenting to Accident and Emergency or on-call junior psychiatrist but excluding patients requiring

mandatory psychiatric admission, those already in contact with the psychiatric services.

(C) St George's: all patients presenting to a sector team, excluding patients in treatment during last 1 year.

(D) Manchester: all patients presenting for admission, excluding patients requiring mandatory admission (section of Mental Health Act (MHA) or clinician judgement).

(E) Birmingham: all seriously ill patients who would normally have been treated in hospital for their acute relapses.

The age range was 16–65 years (75 years for group C). Studies A, B and D excluded patients with a primary diagnosis of drug or alcohol dependence.

It is apparent from the above that no two studies are identical in terms of the patients recruited.

Types of services

The types of services are different. DLP, EIS and Birmingham have special experimental teams set up for the project. St George's and Manchester have routine clinical teams whose work was evaluated in the projects (Table 2.1).

In two services, there have been changes in staffing during collection. The Birmingham study added a 24-on-call system between the first and second reports. The Manchester study has included a limited on-call system and CPN attached to the day hospital (see below).

Patients included in each study

The DLP and Birmingham services included all seriously ill patients presenting for admission. The St George's service also included potential outpatients.

The EIS and Manchester studies excluded patients requiring 'mandatory' admission; the patients included in these studies comprised 58% of all patients presenting for admission at Manchester.

Demographic and diagnostic variables

The different catchment areas and methods of including patients led to different groups of patients being included (Table 2.2).

Table 2.1 Staffing and working hours in five centres in England in which community and hospital services have been compared

	Daily Living Programme	Early Intervention Study	St George's	Manchester	Birmingham
Staff	6 Nurses 1 OT 1 SW 1 Psychiatrist (SR) 1 Secretary	2 CPN 2 SW Psychologist 1 Psychiatrist (Con) 1 Administrator	Sector team	Well-staffed day hospital	1 SW 1 Nurse 1 OT 2 Instructors Psychologist Psychiatrist (Registrar plus 1/2 consultant) 2 CPNs 2 NAs
24-hour on-call	Yes	No	No	No	Yes

CPN: community psychiatric nurse; NA: nursing auxillary; OT: occupational therapist; SR: senior registrar; SW: social worker; Con: consultant.

Table 2.2 *Demographic and diagnostic characteristics of the patients included at the five centres*

	Daily Living programme	Early Intervention Study	St George's	Manchester	Birmingham
Mean Age (years)	34	32	41	43	36
Male(%)	47	40	44	56	43
Single		49	37	42	35
Married		28	38	40	46
S/div/w		23	26	18	19
Non-Caucasians(%)	37	32	8	18	60
First admission (%)	61		25		35
Living alone (%)	38		52		27
Employed(%)	35			48	
Schizophrenia/mania(%)	66	38	35	36	50
Neurotic disorders(%)	12	25	56	27	13

S/div/w: single/divorced/widowed.

The most notable differences are the socio-demographic characteristics of the St George's sample (low proportion of non-Caucasians and high proportion in employment) which are at the opposite end of the spectrum from the DLP.

The high proportion of schizophrenic/manic patients in the DLP and Birmingham studies relate to the selection and severity of illness in the patients recruited.

Severity of illness

The severity of illness included in the studies differed (Table 2.3).

The difference in Brief Psychiatric Rating Scale (BPRS) scores for DLP and St George's indicate the enormous difference between the two groups of patients. They could not be compared in a meta-analysis.

The proportion admitted under section of the Mental Health Act refers to the proportion of potential/actual admissions. For DLP 27% of the patients with severe mental illness requiring immediate admission were being considered for compulsory admission. In the St George's study 44 (25%) of patients were actually admitted and one-quarter were compulsory admissions.

Outcome of experimental and control treatments
Clinical outcome

Table 2.4 illustrates the overall outcome of the four relevant studies. There are difficulties of comparability. The DLP and St George's used BPRS, the EIS used the CPRS, the Manchester study used PSE but the current Manchester study (incomplete) used the CPRS. The interim results are given for comparison.

Significant differences have been reported only at 20 months in the DLP study and 12 weeks in the EIS. The St George's study showed no significant difference at 6 weeks or 1 year. The data for Manchester are taken from the ongoing study (not yet complete) as this has used the CPRS. No significant differences have been found at 12 weeks or 1 year (incomplete results).

Social outcome

The studies used different measures, although the (self-administered) Social Functioning Questionnaire (SFQ) used in the EIS is derived from

Table 2.3 Severity of illness on entry in the five centres

	Daily Living Programme	Early Intervention Study	St George's	Manchester	Birmingham
PSE DAH	5.3		0.8	1.8	3.1
BSO	5.1		1.1	1.1	3.5
SNR	5.9		5.0	4.1	5.69
NSN	12		10.3	9.8	10.4
Total	28.3		18.2		22.72
ID Level 5			26%		16.9%
6			28		20
7			19		29
8			5		21
BPRS	52.2		23		
CPRS		31.5		25	21.64
Mental Health Act (%)	27	0	25(11/44)	0	

BPRS: Basic Psychiatric Rating Score; BSO: Behaviour, Speech and other Syndromes; CPRS: Comprehensive Psychopathological Rating Scale; DAH: Delusions and Hallucinations; NSN: Non-Specific Neurotic Symptoms; SNR: Specific Neurotic Reaction.

Table 2.4 *Comparison of clinical outcome using the Brief Psychiatric Scale (BPRS) or Comprehensive Psychopathological Rating Scale (CPRS) in experimental (community) or control (hospital) groups*

BPRS/ CPRS	DLP		St George's		EIS		Manchester		Birmingham (CPRS)	
	Exp.	Con.	Exp.	Con.	Exp.	Con.	Exp.	Con.	Exp.	Con.
At intake	52	51	7.4	8	33	29	25	24	(22	20)
At 6–11 weeks	39	41	5.5	5.5	21	24	10	7.8		
	NSD		NSD		*P<0.05					
At 12 months	38	40	4	3.6			(10	9)	10.1	9.9
	NSD		NSD				(NSD)		(NSD)	
At 20 months	35	40								
	*P=0.03									

NSD: no significant differences. DLP: Daily Living Programme; EIS: Early Intervention Study; Exp.: experimental; Con.: control.

the Social Functioning Schedule (SFS) used in the St George's study. No significant differences were observed between experimental and control groups in the St George's and EIS and Birmingham studies. In the DLP, the SAS global scale showed significantly greater improvement in the experimental group but only at 20 months. In the Manchester study, the only significant difference favoured the inpatient group at 3 months only; there was no significant difference at 12 months or in the behaviour and burden scales (Table 2.5).

Satisfaction

The satisfaction scores show very clear superiority of home based treatments in DLP and EIS but not in the St George's study (Table 2.6). Manchester did not measure satisfaction.

DLP also measured satisfaction among relatives. There was a significant superiority of home based treatment but not as clear as that demonstrated by the patients. The Birmingham study included relative satisfaction: 43% of the relatives in the experimental group and 23% of the relatives in the control group expressed overall satisfaction with the service ($P < 0.02$).

Bed usage

The differences between home based and control treatments are clearest with regard to bed usage. Table 2.7 shows mean duration of bed usage in each study.

Summary of findings

The overall outcome results are summarised in Figure 2.1. This figure summarises the main results for experimental and control groups of the five relevant studies. The top left hand figure indicates a greater reduction in psychiatric symptoms (i.e. taller columns represent greater change); the experimental group shows a greater change than the control group in two of the five studies (see also Table 2.2). This is also true for social functioning; however, the overall impression in terms of psychiatric symptoms and social functioning is that any difference between experimental and control groups, although statistically significant, is not dramatic. By contrast, the differences in length of inpatient stay (bottom

Table 2.5 Social outcome in the five centres using the Social Adjustment Schedule (SAS), Social Functioning Schedule (SFS), Social Functioning Questionnaire (SFQ) and Social Behaviour Assessment Schedule (SBAS)

Measure	DLP SAS global		St George's SFS		EIS SFQ		Manchester SBAS role		Birmingham	
	Exp.	Con.	Exp.	Con.	Exp.	Con.	Exp.	Con.	Exp.	Con.
At intake	4.5	4.7	19.6	18	11	11	12	14	10	11
At 4 months	3.4	3.6	11.4	12.6	10	10	9	6	6	6
At 11 months	2.9	3.2	13	13.8	NSD		8	7	4	4
At 20 months	2.5	3.1	NSD				NSD		NSD	

NSD (St George's SFS at 4 months); *P=0.03 (DLP SAS global).

Exp.: experimental; Con.: control; NSD: no significant difference. For other abbreviations see Table 2.4.

Table 2.6 *Comparison of patient satisfaction services in experimental and control groups in three centres*

Measure	DLP		St George's		EIS	
	Exp.	Con.	Exp.	Con.	Exp.	Con.
At 3–4 months	25	24	4.9	4.7	25.5	18.9
						*P<0.001
At 11 months	27	22	5.0	5.3		
				NSD		
At 20 months	27	22				
		*P<0.01				

NSD: no significant difference. For other abbreviations see Table 2.4.
DLP also measured satisfaction among relatives. There was a significant superiority of home based treatment but not as clear as for the patients.

left corner of Figure 2.1) are dramatic. Patients treated in community settings consume far fewer bed days than those in standard care.

Follow-up of samples

There is a problem with all these studies which reflects the nature of the patients recruited. Whereas Stein and Test were able to follow up 121 of 122 patients at 1 year, the follow-up rates of the other studies were as follows:

Hoult: 85% at 1 year
DLP: 75% at 20 months
St George's: 66% at 1 year
EIS: 85% at 12 weeks
Manchester: 79% at 1 year.

Can such treatments be generalised?

Our own attempt in Manchester to use the day hospital for acute illness has not been successfully generalised to a second day hospital (Creed *et al.*, 1991*b*). Table 2.8 indicates how the random allocation process differed in the two centres at Manchester and Blackburn.

At Manchester 175 patients were admitted during the study period and of these 35 were successfully engaged in day hospital treatment (six were transferred to inpatient care because they could not be managed in the day hospital.) Assuming another 35 in the inpatient limb, 35 +

Table 2.7 Comparison of mean bed occupancy in experimental and control groups in four centres

Measure	DLP		St George's		EIS		Manchester		Birmingham	
	Exp.	Con.	Exp.	Con.	Exp.	Con.	Exp.	Con.	Exp.	Con.
Mean (SD)	24	106	6.7 (24)	13.7 (25)	1.2	9.3	31 days	36	8 days	59
	*P<0.0001		*P=0.02						p<0.001	

For abbreviations see Table 2.4.

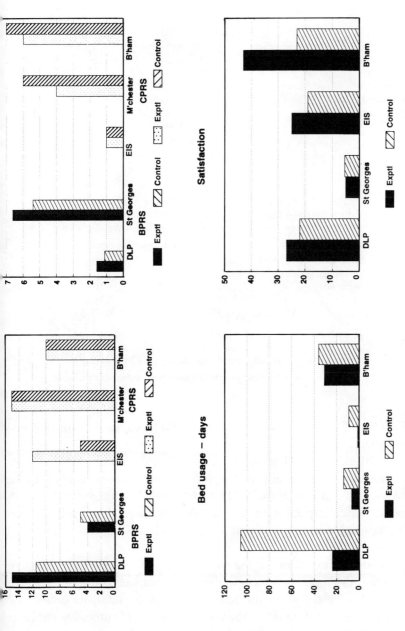

Figure 2.1 Summary of the main results for the experimental and control groups of the five studies.

Table 2.8 *Comparison of recruitment rates in Manchester and Blackburn*

Number of patients	Manchester		Blackburn	
	Inpatient	Day	Inpatient	Day
Allocated	51	51	35	35
Lost after allocation	3	10	3	19
Assessed	48	41	32	19
Engaged in day treatment		35 (6 moved to inpatient)		19

Table 2.9 *Comparison of Nurses; Rating Scale Scores of disturbed behaviour in Manchester and Blackburn studies. A higher score denotes more disturbed behaviour*

Site	Allocation	Median (range)
Manchester	Non-allocated ('too ill')	12 (0–41)
	Randomised (day)	7 (0–22)
	Randomised (inpatient)	6 (0–25)
Blackburn	Non-allocated ('too ill')	11 (0–41)
	Randomised (day)	2.5 (0–12) **
	Randomised (inpatient)	8 (0–27)

35 = 70/175 = 40% of all admissions could be engaged in day hospital treatment.

At Blackburn, 143 patients were admitted overall, only 19 were successfully engaged in day hospital treatment (none needed to be transferred), so 19 + 19 = 38/143 = 26% could be engaged in day treatment. Closer inspection of the data demonstrated that the Blackburn day hospital was not admitting patients with any degree of disturbed behaviour (Table 2.9).

The differences between the two day hospitals, which might account for these discrepancies, include the larger number and more positive approach of the staff in the Manchester day hospital, its brand new building and the distance to the inpatient unit. This probably indicates the enormous training needs of day hospital staff if they are to admit and engage acutely ill patients.

Table 2.10 *Comparison of diagnoses in patients referred to the Early Intervention Service (EIS) in different years*

Measure	1988–89 (%)	1989–90 (%)
Schizophrenia	24	38
Mood disorders	24	32
Neurotic and related	36	25
Substance abuse	12	4
Other	4	1

Table 2.11 *Comparison of diagnoses in Birmingham (Sparkbrook) studies in succeeding years*

	1987–88 (%)		1988–89 (%)	
	Home	Hospital	Home	Hospital
Schizophrenia	37	17	25	23
Manic	21	22	22	35
Depression	26	31.5	45	21
Neurotic and related	–	16.5		
Substance abuse	8	9	9	21
Other	8	2		

Can such treatments be sustained?

The first report of the EIS (Onyett *et al.*, 1990) included 387 patients seen during the first 18 months (January 1988 to mid-1989). The experimental report (1992) included 100 patients (from May 1989 to June 1990). There appears to have been a trend to more severe disorders, at least by diagnosis (Table 2.10).

The Birmingham study has been also been reported twice (Dean & Gadd, 1989, 1990); the second assessment is especially interesting as a 24-hour on-call service was introduced between the two surveys. The diagnostic categories do not change much although there is a trend for fewer patients with schizophrenia and mania, and an increase in the number of depressed patients (Table 2.11).

The first Manchester random allocation study has been followed by a second modified cost-benefit one. This means that admissions to the day hospital have been monitored for nearly 6 years. The effect of an additional CPN to the day hospital further increased severity of illness that can be treated in the day hospital (data not shown).

Conclusion

Data have been presented that compared the experimental and control treatments in five studies. They show that reduction of bed usage is a much clearer result of community treatment than greater improvement of symptoms or social functioning. These results should be thoroughly discussed and understood before policy makers assume that community treatment for acute illness is regarded as 'better' than hospital treatment if we are to overcome Marks' criticism that 'findings from the careful investigations that have been done are usually too slow to disseminate and inform policy making . . . It is also unusual for policy to be tested on a small scale . . . before it is applied nationally, even where such piloting is perfectly practicable and would reduce the chances of making major mistakes that are expensive to correct'.

References

Burns T, Beadsmoore A, Bhat A, Oliver A, Mathers C (1993). A controlled trial of home-based acute psychiatric services. *British Journal of Psychiatry*, **163**: 49–61.

Creed FH, Black D, Anthony P, Osborn M, Thomas P, Tomenson B (1991a). Day hospital for acute psychiatric illness. *British Medical Journal*, **300**: 1033–7.

Creed FH, Black D, Anthony P *et al.* (1991b). Randomised controlled trial of day and inpatient psychiatric treatment. 2. Comparison of two hospitals. *British Journal Psychiatry*, **158**: 183–9.

Dean C, Gadd E (1989). An inner city home treatment service for acute psychiatric patients. *Psychiatric Bulletin*, **13**: 667–9.

Dean C, Gadd EM (1990). Home treatment for acute psychiatric illness. *British Medical Journal*, **301**: 1021–3.

Hoult J (1986). Community care of the acutely mentally ill. *British Journal Psychiatry*, **149**: 137–44.

Merson S, Tyrer P, Onyett S, Lack S, Birkett P, Lynch S, Johnson T (1992). Early intervention in psychiatric emergencies. *Lancet*, **339**: 1311–14.

Muijen M, Marks I, Connolly J, Audini B. (1992). Home based care for patients with severe mental illness. *British Medical Journal*, **304**: 749–54.

National Institute of Mental Health (1991). Caring for people with severe mental disorders: a national plan to improve services. DHHS Publication No. (ADM) 91–1762. Washington DC: Superintendent of Documents US Government Printing Office.

Onyett S, Tyrer P, Connolly J, Malone S, Rennison J, Parslow S, Davey T, Lynch S, Merson S (1990). The Early Intervention Service: the first 18 months of an Inner London demonstration project. *Psychiatric Bulletin*, **14**: 267–9.

Rosen A (1992). Community psychiatry services: will they endure? *Current Opinion in Psychiatry*, **5**: 257–65.

Stein LJ, Test MA (1980). Alternative to mental hospital treatment. 1. Conceptual model treatment program and clinical evaluation. *Archives of General Psychiatry*, **37**: 392–7.

3

Synopsis of the Daily Living Programme for the seriously mentally ill: a controlled comparison of home and hospital based care

ISAAC MARKS

Introduction

Two sources of ambiguity

The subject of this book is the functioning of community care and is mainly concerned with acute psychiatric illness. Ambiguities in this frame of reference require examination to understand the Daily Living Programme (DLP) study discussed below. Such ambiguities reflect universal difficulties in the classification of psychiatric illnesses and their treatments.

The first type of ambiguity concerns the term 'acute'. Does 'acute' mean sudden onset, recent onset, marked severity or all three? Does it include sudden recent onset of severe obsessive–compulsive disorder which can cripple the patient and family as much and for as long as do psychotic disorders? Are we only considering schizophrenia and affective psychosis? Does 'acute' mean a first-ever crisis? Can it mean a new crisis in a chronic illness? Does it include the same patients when they are no longer in crisis? Similar ambiguities also appear if we use the term 'severe mental illness' (SMI) instead of 'acute' mental illness.

Meaningful comparisons across treatment studies require reasonable similarities across their patient samples. Creed's valuable contrast (Chapter 1) showed that in none of the DLP and four other studies presented in this volume did every patient have a diagnosis of schizophrenia or affective psychosis. Following entry to the study only 12% of the DLP patients turned out to have a non-psychotic diagnosis on the Present State Examination (PSE), in contrast to the far higher proportion in the other studies described in this volume. The DLP had a higher proportion of patients with schizophrenia (49%) than did any of the other studies. This point is crucial because in the long run most psychotic patients

29

require a much heavier and continuing therapeutic investment than do neurotic ones, as we will see below.

A second source of ambiguity to keep in mind is the term 'community' treatment. It is not easy to define. Does it only mean home-based treatment? Is community care solely that care which takes place inside the catchment area? Is care in a chronic inpatient ward which is situated inside the catchment area not community care? Do we consider a day hospital to be in the community? If so, is outpatient care a form of community treatment? Does community care also include voluntary services for conditions not usually regarded as SMI. For example the TOP (Triumph Over Phobia) self-exposure groups for anxiety disorders which are spreading in the UK are run by lay leaders and some TOP groups hold their meetings in a room in a hospital; does that mean they are not in community care?

There follows an abbreviated view of the DLP, a controlled study of home based compared to hospital based care. Detailed reports of its preliminary data were published by Muijen *et al.* (1992*a,b*), its first phase results from months 0–20 by Marks *et al.* (1994), a cost–benefit analysis of those results by Knapp *et al.* (1994), the second phase results from months 20–45 by Audini *et al.* (1994) and the mode of clinical working by Connolly *et al.* (unpublished data).

Funding and staffing of the study

The DLP study was carried out in two successive clinical phases which lasted for 62 months overall from intake of the first patient in October 1987 to its closure in December 1992 (Figure 3.1). It was a randomised controlled study which compared home based with in/outpatient care for 189 SMI cases facing emergency admission. The first phase study tracked patient progress for 20 months after entry. In the second phase, from about months 30–45 after entry, DLP care was withdrawn from a randomised half of most of the contactable DLP patients (as in a drug withdrawal study) and patients were followed for a further 15 months. Most of the original trial entrants were followed over both phases of the study for nearly 3 years. The bulk of the data in this chapter refer to the first phase. Results of the withdrawal phase are still being analysed.

The arduous clinical work of the DLP arm throughout both phases was led by consultant psychiatrist, Dr J. Connolly, with a senior registrar a and a nurse manager. In this phase most of the team were nurses; a nurse was replaced serially by a social worker for 14 months only and

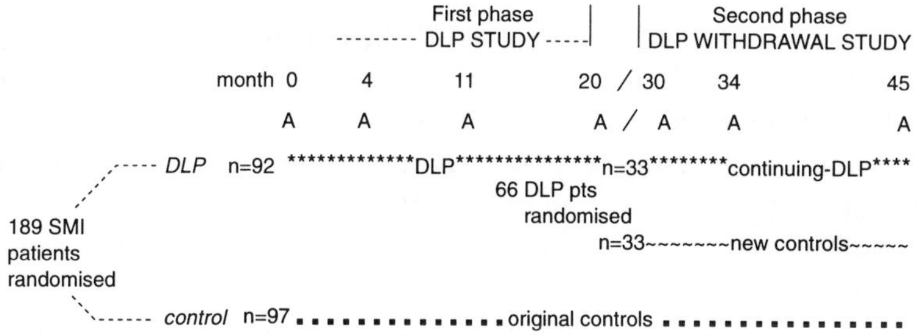

```
                          First phase     |   |    Second phase
                      --------- DLP STUDY ----|   | DLP WITHDRAWAL STUDY

       month  0      4       11          20  /  30      34                45

                A       A       A           A  /  A       A                 A

     ,----- DLP   n=92 *************DLP**************n=33********continuing-DLP****
    /--                                      66 DLP pts
   /                                         randomised
 189 SMI                                          n=33~~~~~~~new controls~~~~~
 patients
 randomised
   \                                                       .
    \------ control  n=97 ·············· · original controls ··············· · ·
```

First phase DLP STUDY

189 SMI patients facing emergency admission from London inner city catchment area randomised to have 20 months of:

HOME-BASED CARE (+INPATIENT SPELLS AS NEEDED) *DLP community care*   (n=92)

or

INPATIENT FOLLOWED BY OUTPATIENT CARE *control* standard hospital care   (n=97)

Second phase DLP WITHDRAWAL STUDY

At 20 months post-entry, 66* DLP patients randomised to 15 months of:

CONTINUING HOME-BASED CARE   *DLP* (n=33)

or

OUT/INPATIENT CARE AS NEEDED control standard hospital care   (n=33)

*criteria for inclusion in withdrawal study
    PSE SMI category
    patient agrees to followup
    still being seen regularly by DLP team

Figure 3.1 Design of the study.

two occupational therapists. In the second (withdrawal) phase there were substantial changes in the clinical staff although the representation of disciplines was similar.

Professor Isaac Marks was responsible for the small amount of training in the DLP arm in the first phase (there was none in the second phase) and for the extensive evaluation of both phases. Professor Martin Knapp and Dr Jeni Beecham carried out the cost–benefit analysis of the first phase.

Clinical work

All patients were first seen during a crisis in which a doctor not involved in the DLP and usually staffing the 24-hour Emergency Clinic thought immediate admission was indicated for serious mental illness.

If patients were randomised to DLP then their care became largely home based, although 88% of them also had at least one inpatient spell at some stage in the first phase, most commonly at the start and often subsequently. Patients who drew control care had the usual inpatient followed by outpatient care offered at the time at the Maudsley Hospital; few facilities were available then for outreach if control patients defaulted.

The clinical team giving home based DLP care was specially set up for the purpose and there were important changes in staff during the life of the study. Most care was given by day but staff were on a 24-hour duty bleep rota of availability on the telephone. Although seldom used, this telephone availability round the clock in an emergency was reassuring to many patients and relatives. Until 28 months into the study the DLP staff participated in any inpatient spells of care and were responsible for discharge. The care was largely problem-oriented, with the definition of problems and goals to deal with them and the monitoring of how those were being met, usually being at the core of the care plan. Progress on these problems and goals was audited regularly. Some staff resisted training in and the use of this approach.

DLP care did not include systematic family work to reduce high expressed emotion; nor did the DLP team systematically use behavioural methods to reduce symptoms. This was because at the time the study began in 1987 the evidence for the value of these approaches was limited and training in them was too early for incorporation.

The sample

Of all cases, 65% were would-be new admissions and the rest were re-admissions. The DLP group contained a non-significant excess of first admissions to any psychiatric hospital; 27% of all patients entered the trial on a Section of the Mental Health Act. The great majority of baseline features were balanced across the DLP and control groups: mean age was 34 years, 49% were male, 40% lived with no support (alone or single with young children) and only 35% had a paid job. Ethnic background was similar to that of the local catchment area population: 63% British/Irish, 23% Afro-Caribbean (only 5% more than the area norm), 14% other.

At trial entry the would-be admitting psychiatrist in the Emergency Clinic thought that every patient had SMI. The PSE performed shortly after trial entry, however, yielded a diagnosis of 49% schizophrenia,

19% depression, 17% mania, 12% neurosis and 3% unclassifiable. At baseline, DLP and control patients had severe psychopathology.

Outcome of the first phase (months 0–20)

The outcome was similar whether patients had been first admissions or re-admissions at entry into the trial. DLP patients in the first phase used a striking 80% fewer inpatient bed days than did controls. This was evident from months 3 to 20. However, as discussed below, home based treatment was not the sole factor which reduced the number of bed days used. We should also note that the DLP patients had as many admissions as the controls. The 'revolving door' continued but the number of inpatient beds needed fell because the duration of inpatient spells was sharply reduced with far more time spent outside hospital.

With regard to clinical outcome, the few between-group significant differences consistently favoured DLP over control patients, mainly at 20 months (Table 3.1). At that point DLP were slightly but significantly superior to control patients on the BPRS, specific neurotic symptoms of the PSE, social adjustment globally, with parents, and on daily living skills, and tended to be better than controls on the Global Adjustment Scale (GAS). It is remarkable that it took nearly 20 months before home based care showed significant clinical superiority. Even then that superiority was very limited, with most patients remaining unemployed and needing continuing monitoring and assertive outreach.

Why did the limited clinical and social superiority of home based care take 20 months to become detectable? One possibility is that it took the DLP team perhaps a year to know how to operate, what skills needed to be trained and to train in such skills, albeit far too little (see below).

DLP patients were distinctly more satisfied with their treatment than were controls. This greater satisfaction appeared earlier than the clinical gains, from 11 months onwards. To a lesser extent DLP patients' relatives were also more satisfied with the treatment than were control patients' relatives, even though (or perhaps because?) DLP patients had spent far less time away from them as inpatients. Only 53% of patients were living with their families at 20 months and such patients often refused to allow relatives to be evaluated, but their satisfaction ratings did match the superiority of DLP care in improving relationships with parents. The advantage of home based care was thus obtained without obviously burdening the family. Satisfaction and clinical outcome are independent measures, however, as we will see later.

Table 3.1. *Outcome of the first phase*

	DLP superiority to controls	
	20 months	34–45 months
No. of inpatient days	80% less	(more)[a]
Clinical		
BPRS	Significant	NS
PSE specific neurotic symptoms	Significant	Significant
Social adjustment		
Global	Significant	NS
With parents	Significant	NS
Daily living skills	Significant	NS
Global adjustment	Trend	NS
Satisfaction of		
Patient	Significant	Significant
Relative	Significant	Significant
Cost of care	Significant	

BPRS: Basic Psychiatric Rating Score; PSE, Present State Examination.
Significant: $P < 0.05$ or better; Trend: P 0.1; NS: not significant.
[a] Continuing Daily Living Programme (DLP) group used more inpatient days than did new-control group.

As the DLP name indicates, DLP patients were trained in daily living skills. This showed up in their greater improvement compared with control patients in daily living skills at 20 months. Perhaps this made DLP patients easier to live with. Perhaps too, the longer time that controls spent as inpatients, during which time their families had little contact with them or their clinicians, had alienated control patients from their relatives and begun a process of institutionalisation. DLP patients had more chance to maintain social ties as they were away from home for far less time and the DLP team gave frequent support to their families.

Many think that disturbed patients do better in a ward that is monitored 24 hours a day. We found this not to be so. The slightly better outcome from, and preference of patients and their relatives for, well-supported care outside hospital meshes with other advances in the care of acute and chronic health care problems. Women often prefer to give birth at home. It is now common to have hospital day surgery with aftercare while living at home. Chronic renal patients increasingly dialyse themselves at home.

Throughout the 20 months of the first phase, DLP care cost significantly less than did control care. Professor Knapp summarises the cost–benefit analysis in Chapter 10. The important point here is that the greater consumer satisfaction and marginally better clinical and social outcome which were obtained with home based care throughout the first phase cost no more than did the traditional alternative hospital based care. In fact, the reverse was the case; not only in the initial crisis phase but also from months 11 to 20.

The DLP results over the first 20 months in an inner city UK area are in line with those in previous controlled studies in the more affluent Madison and Sydney settings (which lasted 12 months). In all three studies the proportion of bed days saved was about 80% and home based care cost less than hospital based care. Although our scales differed from those in the Madison study, the directions of change were the same. Several of our scales were similar to those in the Sydney study; on the Global Assessment Scale (GAS), Brief Psychiatric Rating Scale (BPRS) and PSE the percentage of improvement was very similar. Gains in social adjustment and in patient and relative satisfaction were comparable. One difference between the DLP and the other studies was the 20-month delay before superiority of home to hospital based care emerged on clinical and social scales.

Preliminary results of the second (partial withdrawal) phase

The main report of the findings from this phase is by Audini *et al.* (1994). The results are chastening. The mean number of inpatient bed days became the same across the continuing DLP and new control groups, although only a minority of patients had an inpatient phase. Continuing DLP patients and their relatives remained more satisfied than the new control counterparts from whom DLP care was withdrawn (Figure 3.2) but this greater satisfaction was not reflected by greater clinical or social improvement on most of the measures. Consumer satisfaction may be more a reflection of staff visits to patients' and relatives' homes rather than a reflection of what those visits achieved.

The only scale on which the superiority at 20 months of home based care was maintained through the second phase was PSE non-specific neurotic symptoms and this was not matched by any superiority on the comparable BPRS subscores for anxiety and depression. During months 30 to 45 both the continuing DLP patients and the new controls gradually lost some of the gains they had shown at 20 months after initial

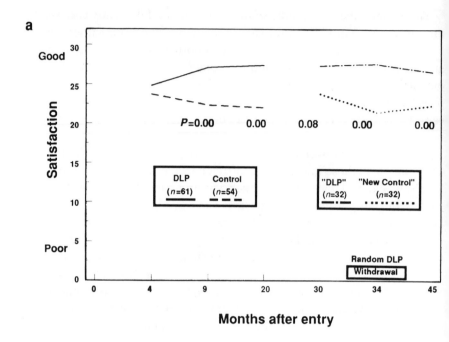

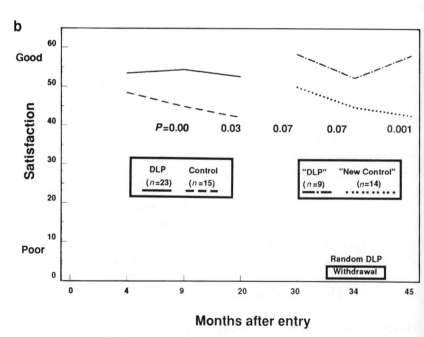

Figure 3.2 Results of the second (partial withdrawal) phase of the trial showing (a) client's and (b) relative's satisfaction.

Table 3.2 *Limitations of home based care*

Daily Living Programme care did not:
Cure serious mental illness
Lower the death rate
Stop the 'revolving door'
Stop indefinitely the continuing need for:
Heavy staff input
Assertive outreach

entry. Also, in the Madison study, patients gradually lost their gains after community care stopped at 14 months after entry.

Why did patients who continued with DLP care through the second phase nevertheless start to worsen? Continuing DLP care in the second phase (months 30–45) differed from that in the first phase (months 0–20). Five differences can be identified in DLP first- versus second-phase care and perhaps one difference in control first- versus second-phase care.

For DLP care during the second phase compared with the first phase: (1) the DLP suffered major staff changes, (2) there was no training in problem-oriented care, (3) there was attenuation of the problem-oriented way of working, (4) DLP staff were no longer allowed by the hospital to be responsible for discharge from any inpatient phases which DLP patients might have, (5) relevant to (4), DLP staff were demoralised from (a) the legacy of a media and hospital audit ordeal in the third year of the study (see below) and (b) prolonged uncertainty about how long second-phase funding would continue. Another difference is that control care in the second phase may have altered partly due to the first-phase DLP results having been fed back to the hospital.

Effective home based care is hard to organise, is vulnerable to many factors and needs careful training and regular clinical audit if the problem-oriented mode of working is to be sustained.

What DLP care did not achieve

The significant advantages of home over hospital based care must be put in perspective. The fashion for community care makes it easy to forget four strong limitations (Table 3.2).

Firstly, home based care did not cure SMI. Although home based care was preferred throughout and was superior to and less costly than hospital based care from months 0 to 20, the clinical and social gains it produced were distinctly limited. Not only the DLP but also the control groups improved significantly by month 4 and remained so until 20 months, although overall each group contained relapsing patients. Despite their clinical and social improvement, only a quarter of patients had a paid job at 20 months which is less than the 35% at the time of entry. Not a few patients remained very disturbed and dependent or refused medication through to the end of the study. Six (two DLP, four control) patients had to be transferred to long-stay inpatient care by the 20-month rating.

The second failure stems from the first. Home based care did not stop the revolving door of re-admissions. Although the duration of inpatient stays of DLP patients was far less than for control patients as long as the DLP team had responsibility for those stays, the number of admissions did not change. Good community care requires some beds for brief crisis admissions, preferably under the responsibility of the community team.

The third failure also stems from the first. Home based care did not stop the continuing need of SMI patients for heavy staff input and assertive outreach year after year. This was highlighted when the DLP matched staff time invested to clinical progress achieved. To maintain asylum functions in good community care, key workers must coordinate many different community resources and regularly visit defaulters. This drains staff time.

The DLP staff's mean number of clinical contacts and hours per case was about 25 in the first month after trial entry, dropping to an asymptote of eight contacts and 5 hours per month from month 6 onwards time per contact being about 40 minutes. Psychotic cases required far more time than did the minority of neurotic ones. With unresponsive patients the load never stopped, year in and year out, taking hundreds of hours of staff time a year, with more during crises and less between, but never zero. Although a problem-oriented approach seems to reduce DLP time needed, the burden on carers remains great in tough cases.

The heavy load from SMI patients contrasts starkly with the far lighter demand on staff time made, say, by the behavioural treatment of anxiety disorders (Marks, 1992). This is not because all anxiety disorders are less severely disabling than is SMI. Far from it – they can cripple sufferers and their families just as much as SMI does and hardly deserve their occasional label of 'minor' psychiatric illness.

The contrast in staff time needed stems rather from differences in the efficacy of current treatment methods for different conditions. With only 8–15 hours of clinician time spent giving appropriate behaviour therapy, even when symptoms are severe and chronic, most anxiety disorder patients show major and enduring improvement in symptoms, work and social adjustment and the treatment is then largely finished. This is not so with chronic SMI. Even our best medication and psychosocial treatments together still yield only modest gains in chronic schizophrenia or manic–depressive illness; these disorders need much organisation and staff time, although the effort does seem worth while.

It took time for DLP staff to learn what might be realistically achieved, to help without inducing undue dependency and to persist but not perseverate with rejecting patients. Staff had to specify in advance the goals hoped for from each contact with patients and others and how they fitted into the overall care plan. After each contact appraisal was made of what had been done and what to do next. Unfocused and ineffective care was changed. Waste of time and resources was lessened by recording the duration and type of each contact and what was achieved, totalling all the hours that staff had devoted to a patient's care by a given date and matching those hours against the clinical gains achieved by then. This is the problem-oriented approach.

The final limitation of home based care is certainly not the least one. Home based care did not reduce the number of deaths in this high-risk group of patients. Deaths from self-harm over the 20 months after entry were three in the DLP and two in the control group and a DLP patient murdered a neighbour's daughter. In the second phase after 20 months there was another suicide, in an ex-DLP case who had recently become a control. An original control case killed herself 4 years after entry. Thus, 4 years after the 189 patients entered the study, seven were dead from self-harm (three DLP, three controls and one in transition between the two conditions). Two more cases were dead by then from natural causes: one DLP case died from cervical cancer and another from a subdural haematoma after a fall.

The high suicide risk of SMI patients is well known (Cohen *et al.*, 1990; Anderson *et al.*, 1991). In the follow-up to the Madison study good community support failed to prevent several suicides. In that study, completed suicide was predicted not by the last mental state evaluated prior to the suicide but rather by the baseline severity at entry into the study. In the Bethlem-Maudsley Hospital as a whole outside our study we found that there was a suicide on average about every 6 weeks in inpatients and recently discharged patients. We could find no record of

Isaac Marks

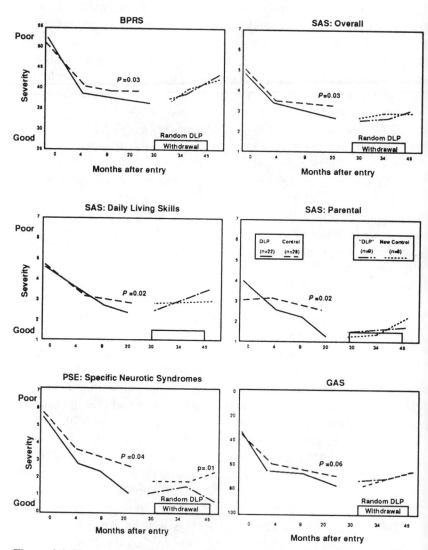

Figure 3.3 Home versus hospital care. (——) DLP, *n* = 92. (–––) Control, *n* = 97. (–·–·) 'DLP', *n* = 33. (····) 'New control', *n* = 33. 0.03, 0.02 etc. are significance of ANCOVA of between group differences for months 0–20 and 30–45.

he suicide rate of similar SMI patients treated in other hospitals with which we could compare the overall Maudsley rate. The frequency of suicides in hospital and in the community makes one wonder about the possibility of achieving the 'Health of the Nation' target of suicide reduction just by intensive psychiatric treatment and support without appropriate wider social measures.

A murder media ordeal and ensuing natural experiment

The tragic murder of a baby by a DLP patient only had a brief mention in a local paper at the time but 14 months later there was a massive outcry in the national media and a Parliamentary debate which almost led to closure of the DLP study (this crisis began in the week we had just written to the Department of Health (DoH) for our final year's funding; continuing DoH support through this crisis was vital in allowing us to complete the study). In the wake of the media ordeal a Hospital Audit was made of the DLP team's work. It exonerated the staff from blame and praised its work but ruled that DLP staff cease to be responsible for the timing of discharge of DLP patients from any inpatient phase which was needed.

This Audit ruling produced a valuable natural experiment. Once the DLP staff had to relinquish to ward staff the responsibility for discharge from hospital, the average length of such crisis hospital stays trebled. Moreover, in the second phase of the project (months 30–45), carried out entirely under this rule imposed after the Hospital Audit, the number of bed days used by the continuing DLP and the new control groups became almost identical, having trebled from 18 in the first phase to 52 in the continuing DLP group and diminished among controls from 72 to 51 days.

Home based care per se was thus not the only factor which reduced the number of bed days during the project's first phase (months 0–20). An additional factor decreasing the length of inpatient stay was that for most of months 0 to 20 the community team had been responsible also for any inpatient discharge, so increasing the continuity of care between community and inpatient phases. Ensuring such continuity is crucial in the planning of services.

Training in home based care

The DLP staff's limited training in community care deserves mention. At the time the DLP study began in 1987 there was no systematic training programme for care of the SMI anywhere, so we had to boot-strap our staffs training. Our senior staff had several exchange visits with Madison staff, whose model we were trying to emulate, and had some interaction with Dr Hoult who had replicated that model in Sydney. Our having no training resources meant that DLP staff had very limited training in problem and goal oriented care. For reasons given earlier, the DLP team did not have systematic training in family work for that half of our patients who were living with their families, nor did they have good training in the behavioural treatment of psychotic symptoms.

The lack of a training programme in problem centred community care for SMI was a major problem in the DLP. This is remedied by the Thorn course to train nurses in London and Manchester. Major components of this course are the problem centred training and manual which was evolved during the DLP study, the family work and symptom management pioneered by Leff and Tarrier, respectively and the regular audit of patient outcome. From these a curriculum and audit method will soon be available for further centres and professions. The advent of staff who are well trained in problem centred community care for SMI should hasten the spread of such care in the UK. This might reduce the real danger of untrained community workers 'owning' patients and preventing them from getting helpful treatment because of, say, undue staff hostility to medication or inattention to proper case management.

The DLP study has raised questions about how much the gain from home based care in the first phase was due to its:

site of care being home based
problem centred focus of care
teaching of daily living skills
assertive follow-up
community staff remaining responsible for any inpatient phase
keyworker coordinating total care across different agencies (case management)
24-hour availability of staff on the telephone
regular audit of progress
other care components.

It is clear from the natural experiment noted above that continuity of care arising from the community team remaining responsible for discharge from any inpatient periods of care during crises is essential if those spells are to be kept short. Such continuity is also likely to improve care overall.

The increase in bed days used during the second phase of the study might also be partly attributable to staff difficulties at that time which led to continuing DLP care becoming less problem centred with less regular audit of progress, as well as no longer including responsibility for inpatient spells. Second-phase staff did continue to carry out home based care, to be available on the telephone round the clock, and to practise assertive outreach.

The DLP has now ceased its work at the Maudsley but a successor District Service in the Nunhead sector has built in several aspects of the DLP care: 24-hour access by patients and relatives to staff on the telephone, control by the community team over their own beds, assertive outreach and liaison with community agencies (Strathdee & Thornicroft, 1992). Problem oriented care is not a focus.

The Thorn training in community care which partly grew out of the DLP study is leading to a demand for such training. Before investment mushrooms in such training and it becomes backed by policy, it may be wise to carry out a randomised controlled study of whether patients cared for by staff who have had such training do better than patients cared for by staff without such training. Such a study could involve both the London and the Manchester sites in which Thorn training takes place, which would yield 24 trainees per year. A study of this kind would extend the valuable work of Brooker and Butterworth which was non-randomised, did not focus on problem centred case management and concerned only patients with schizophrenia who were living with their families and so constitute only about a quarter of the kinds of patients treated by Thorn nurses.

Thorn training has four main components: (1) a problem oriented focus, (2) behavioural management of symptoms, (3) family work (applicable to about a quarter of all SMI patients in the UK), and (4) regular audit of progress. The main outcome areas are clinical and social progress, patient and relative satisfaction and keyworker cost to obtain these outcomes. For future studies of this and other kinds it would be helpful to derive, from the arduous measurement batteries used in research studies so far, more streamlined outcome indicators in SMI which are easy enough for regular staff to use in routine clinical audit. 'Quick and dirty' audit measures can be made reliable. They could help to sustain and disseminate high quality in community care.

References

Anderson C, Connelly J, Johnstone EC, Owens DGC (1991). Disabilities and circumstances of schizophrenic patients: a follow-up study. V. Cause of death. *British Journal of Psychiatry* **159** (Suppl. 13): 30–3.

Audini B, Marks IM, Lawrence RE, Connolly J, Watts V (1994). Home-based vs in/outpatient care for serious mental illness: phase II of a controlled study. *British Journal of Psychiatry* **165**: 204–21.

Cohen L.J, Test MA, Brown RL (1990). Suicide and schizophrenia: data from a prospective community treatment study. *American Journal of Psychiatry*, **147**: 602–7.

Knapp M, Beecham J, Koutsogeorgopoulou V, Hallan A, Fenyo A, Marks IM, connolly J, Audini B (1994). Service use and costs of home-based vs hospital based care for people with serious mental illness. *British Journal of Psychiatry* (in press).

Marks IM (1992). Innovations in mental health care delivery. *British Journal of Psychiatry*, **160**: 589–97.

Marks IM, Connolly J, Muijen M, Audini B, McNamee G, Lawrence RE (1994). Home-based versus hospital-based care for people with serious mental illness. *British Journal of Psychiatry* **165**: 179–94.

Muijen M, Marks IM, Connolly J, Audini B, McNamee G (1992*a*). The Daily Living Program: preliminary comparison of community versus hospital based treatment for the seriously mentally ill facing emergency admission. *British Journal of Psychiatry*, **160**: 379–84.

Muijen M, Marks IM, Connolly J, Audini B (1992*b*). Home based care versus standard hospital based care for the severely mentally ill: short-term outcome. *British Medical Journal*, **304**: 749–54.

Strathdee G, Thornicroft G (1992). Community sectors for needs-led mental health services. In: Thornicroft G, Brewin C, Wing J (eds) *Measuring Mental Health Needs*, chap. 8, Gaskell, London.

4
Evaluation of a complete community service
CHRISTINE DEAN

Introduction

The research in Sparkbrook, Birmingham, differs from the others in this volume in that it was not a randomised controlled trial but an evaluation of a total service. An audit of the service has been performed over several years and a research project has just been completed which is a comparison of Sparkbrook with another total service; Grad & Sainsbury (1968) used a similar design. This design has the disadvantage that the two samples being compared may have different characteristics but it has the advantage that one element of a service is not being picked out and compared with another. It is, for instance, rather artificial to compare inpatient care with day care because in clinical practice a range of treatment options are available. The Sparkbrook service has been running for 6 years and details have been reported elsewhere (Dean & Gadd 1990).

Background

Sparkbrook is a small inner city, deprived electoral ward with a population of 25 725, a Jarman score of +62 and an unemployment rate of 30% (at October 1991). Over 50% of the population are from New Commonwealth or Pakistan (1981 census).

The Resource centre which is situated in the middle of the locality is the focus for all activities. It provides day facilities for approximately 30 people a day: the services provided are a combination of those which would normally be expected in a day hospital and in a day centre. There is a drop-in facility with a relaxed, unstructured, 'cafe-type' atmosphere for people with long-term disability. Users are able to get a free bus pass if they attend several days a week and this enhances their social life as it

45

means that they can also visit other people. Users attending the drop-in centre also get a free meal, in recognition of the poor financial state of many of them. They can join in the other more structured activities if they want to and these include sessions of the usual range of practical and psychotherapeutic activities. On one day a week, there is a special Asian women's group and two members of staff collect the women in a minibus. The psychiatric outpatient and nurses' clinics are now held in the resource centre. Users are also seen as emergencies outside the clinic times, either at their own request or at the request of their general practitioner or other professional. There is a group which is specifically for Caribbean men, while Asian and Caribbean music is played and Asian and Caribbean food provided at some time each week in the centre. The special occasions on the Asian, Caribbean and English calendars are all celebrated.

The current staffing of the centre is shown in Table 4.1; the staff provide all the mental health services to the community, apart from the inpatient services. The combined team have a caseload in excess of 450 of whom 150 have severe long-term disability. The building is owned and run by social services, who also provide the centre's non-staff budget for food, trips and other items of expenditure. Both social services and health services staff are based at the centre. This has many advantages because it means that there is one point of access to the services and users can obtain advice about benefits, housing, occupation and health all under the same roof; this avoids the forced choice between health and social care. All the staff work in the community as well as in the centre and there is a rota to ensure that at least one person is in the centre (in the drop-in area) at any one time. The out-of-hours rota is provided by the community psychiatric and home treatment nurses. Five of the current staff speak Asian languages and it is a policy to assess patients at their initial presentation in their own first language.

The home treatment service was set up as an alternative to hospital admission for people with serious acute psychiatric illness which, in a traditional service, would have resulted in an admission to hospital. The service accepts referrals of people known to the service from any source: general practitioner, health visitor, patient, relative, etc. New referrals are referred by their general practitioner. Urgent referrals are seen by a nurse and a doctor as soon as possible and certainly on the day of referral; in the majority of cases, the patients are assessed initially by at least one member of staff who speaks their language. Thereafter, the staff have a mixed case load but always there is the benefit of advice from

Table 4.1 *Current staffing for the centre*

Social services staff (FTE)[a]	Health service staff (FTE)
Manager (1)	Deputy manager (1)
Instructors (2)	Occupational therapist (1)
Receptionist (1)	Psychologist (0.6)
Community worker (1)	Psychology technician (0.4)
Social worker (2)	Medical secretary (1)
Social work assistant (0.2)	Community psychiatric nurses (3)
Domestic (0.7)	Home treatment nurses (2)
	Nursing auxiliaries (2)
	For nurse on-call (1.2)
	Consultant (0.6)
	Registrar (1)

[a] Full-time equivalent.

someone who speaks the appropriate language if this is required. All the staff carry a limited repertoire of drugs (thioridazine, chlorpromazine, haloperidol, lofepramine, procyclidine, zuclopenthixol acetate), so that initial treatment can be started immediately if this is required. If the patient is regarded as suitable for 'home treatment' he/she has a full 'work up', as if in hospital, with a full history, written case summary and physical examination. The continuation sheets, on which all professionals record their visits, are left in the patient's house together with a medication card and instructions about how to contact the nurse who is available 24 hours a day. For the first few days staff may visit several times a day and may administer the medication if there is a suicide risk or a risk of non-compliance.

At the time of discharge from home treatment, all patients have a discharge plan and they are followed up at outpatient clinics which are run at the resource centre or visited on a regular basis at home if they are not able to attend. They and their relatives are asked to contact us immediately if there are any early signs of relapse. Patients are also offered whatever service they require from the centre; drop-in facility, group activities, social work help, etc. People who are known to the service who have serious long-term disability are visited at home if they fail to turn up for their clinic appointment or for treatment; this work is often done by the on-call team in an evening or at weekends.

The home treatment team also provide a service for people admitted to hospital following a suicide attempt. They (usually a nurse and doctor) assess the person in hospital and decide whether it is necessary to transfer the patient to the psychiatric hospital or to home treatment. Quite frequently, they take the person home from the hospital and make sure that he/she is able to cope in the home environment even if not put on home treatment, or home treatment may be instituted for a few days. With this system and the availability of 24-hour support, very few suicidal patients require admission to hospital.

The community worker has the sole task of helping the users with employment and training. He/she runs job clubs, trains people for interviews and supports them initially if they are successful in obtaining a job or getting on a course. He/she runs seminars for employers to educate them about psychotic disorder and visits the local places of employment to encourage employers to take on service users. He/she studies job advertisements for those which are only for a few hours a week; these jobs are not popular with people who are not on invalidity benefits because they can obtain a higher income on unemployment benefit. He/she has been very successful at getting people into employment.

There is also a variety of leisure opportunities, e.g. day trips in the mini bus, football and snooker matches, an evening social club (visiting restaurants, the cinema, etc.) and a Sunday club. One night a week, they have the opportunity to use all the facilities at the local leisure centre. There is a designated forum for organising leisure activities for the Birmingham health district. Some users go on holidays with the staff for weekends or for a week at home or abroad. There is a music club for people who want to play music. All the staff play a part in these activities. The team as a whole and the social worker and assistant in particular offer help with benefits and housing whereas some team members, usually the nursing auxiliaries and instructors, help with the shopping, household management and budgeting. For those who need it, there are facilities for bathing and shaving and for doing their laundry.

Two carers' groups were established: one for relatives and friends who speak English and one for those who speak Asian languages. The latter was not popular as the Asian families prefer to be supported at home. The English-speaking group meets monthly. Sometimes the staff (several of whom have had training in family therapy) work with families on a sessional basis, either at home or at the centre.

The team also provides a service to Trinity night shelter for the homeless. A doctor and a nurse visit once a week and the community team are available to the staff at the Shelter and also provide support to the nurse who works specifically with the homeless.

There is a process of continuous audit and assessment of consumer satisfaction at Main Street. Every 6 months there is a survey about what people like about the centre, what activities they find enjoyable and useful and what they do not like but would like to see improved. Every 6 months, the staff have a planning day to which some users are invited. The results of the survey are presented at this meeting and in the light of this information the services for the next 6 months are planned. Detailed targets and objectives for the centre are set and these are monitored weekly. In this way, the activities of the centre are kept flexible and responsive to the changing needs of the users.

There is an adult carer scheme in Birmingham which is one where ordinary families take someone with long-term mental illness into their own home. A coordinator employed by social services supports these families and screens new families. It has proved a very successful scheme for a number of people in Sparkbrook who have long-term disability.

In addition to the community facilities, the service uses six acute beds. Unfortunately, there are no staffed long-term or rehabilitation facilities and two patients have been in the ward for 2–3 years. The inpatient beds are very much part of the service. Staff who know patients who have been admitted maintain contact with them in the hospital. The consultant is responsible for the patient in hospital as well as the community and when the person leaves the hospital they are usually taken home by the home treatment nurses and visited for a while after discharge.

These are two employing agencies of the staff at the Centre. This causes difficulties in the management structure with health service staff being responsible to social services staff and vice versa. The manager of the Centre reports to two people, one health and one social services manager, which is unsatisfactory.

Home treatment is provided as an alternative to inpatient care when this is appropriate. Initially Sparkbrook was the only locality providing this kind of service in Birmingham which made medical cover out-of-hours difficult. The sustainability of this kind of service depends on the medical cover being provided as part of the standard district duty rota.

The service has been successful in providing a service to South Asian and Afro-Caribbean people; over 50% of the outpatients, 66% of the home treatment cases and 50% of the inpatients are of Asian or Afro-caribbean origin, which is very similar to the proportion in the general population (50.5%, 1981 census).

The impression of the staff in Sparkbrook over the years of providing a local service is that the number of people relapsing with acute episodes of illness severe enough to require hospital and home treatment has fallen.

Christine Dean

Table 4.2 *Numbers of previous admissions of all patients treated by home treatment or inpatient treatment*

	1987–88	1988–89	1989–90
No previous admissions	26	34	31
Previous admissions			
1–5	46	50	33
6–25	20	15	10

Table 4.2 shows the details of all admissions over a 3-year period. The numbers of people with no previous admissions are fairly static as one might expect. The group who have most reduction in their severe acute episodes are the so called 'revolving door' patients who have had many previous admissions. This is encouraging; it could be because people with long-term disability can refer themselves to the service, they are encouraged to watch out for early warning signs and they are not afraid to present with early symptoms because they know they will not necessarily be admitted to hospital.

Good Practices in Mental Health (Patmore & Weaver 1991, 1992) also evaluated the Sparkbrook service along with five other Department of Health and Social Security (DHSS) multi-agency community schemes. The Sparkbrook service (Team A in the report) was the most successful at targeting people with serious mental illness; 70% of those attending the Resource Centre (outpatients were not included) came into this category.

A study comparing the Sparkbrook service with that of the neighbouring electoral ward Small Heath was recently completed (Dean *et al.*, 1993). Small Heath is served by a different health authority which has similar demographic characteristics to Sparkbrook with 43% of the population from New Commonwealth or Pakistan. Small Heath is not as socially deprived: Jarman score +52.7 compared with Sparkbrook which has a Jarman score (1983) of +62 and 22.8% unemployment at October 1991 compared with 30% in Sparkbrook. The study began in January 1990, 3 years after the establishment of the community service. Between January 1990 and February 1991 all people (aged 16–65 years) living in Sparkbrook and Small Heath who had an illness severe enough to require admission to hospital or home treatment were included in this study. The patients and their relatives were assessed on a number of occasions (Table 4.3).

Table 4.3 *Sparkbrook versus Small Heath study: methods of assessment and time scale*

Method of assessment	Duration	Weeks	Years
Present State Examination	Initially		1
Syndrome checklist	Initially (from medical notes at admission)		
Comprehensive Psychiatric Rating Scale	Completed weekly for 4 weeks		1
Morningside Rating Scale	Completed weekly for 6 weeks		1
Burden Questionnaire (Hoult & Reynolds, 1985)	Initially	4	1
Satisfaction Questionnaire (Hoult & Reynolds, 1985)		4	1
Social Behaviour Assessment Schedule (SBAS)	Initially	4	1
General Hospital Questionnaire (carer)	Initially	4	1
Patients' demography, clinical, social and forensic details	Initially	4	1
Relatives' demography and contact with services	Initially	4	1

The Sparkbrook and Small Heath samples were not different in terms of age, sex or marital status. Thirty-four (49%) Sparkbrook patients had had previous admissions compared with 25 (45%) Small Heath patients. Nineteen (27.5%) Sparkbrook patients had had previous compulsory admissions compared with 12 (21.8%) Small Heath patients. There was no difference between groups in terms of severity of illness (PSE score and subscale scores) or diagnosis (Table 4.4).

Twenty-four (35%) of the Sparkbrook group received some inpatient treatment during the initial episode. The Sparkbrook group had an average of 8 days in hospital in the first admission compared with 59 days in the Small Heath group. During the first year the Sparkbrook group had an average of 20.6 days compared with 67.9 in the Small Heath group.

There was no difference between the two groups in terms of the three scales, disturbed behaviour, objective burden and social performance on the Social Behaviour Assessment Schedule (SBAS), but there was a difference in the relatives' distress. The relatives' distress due to burden and due to social performance of the person in treatment was less in

Table 4.4 *PSE scores and diagnosis at the initial assessment*

PSE scores (SD)	Sparkbrook ($n=65$)[a]	Small Health ($n=51$)[a]
Initial mean PSE total score (SD)	22.724 (13.33)	20.636 (15.154)
Initial DAH Score: mean (SD)	3.086 (4.635)	3.205 (5.232)
Initial BSO Score: mean (SD)	3.534 (3.643)	3.705 (4.811)
SNS Score: mean (SD)	5.69 (5.494)	5.136 (5.161)
NSN Score: mean (SD)	10.414 (7.516)	8.591 (8.070)
ICD diagnosis: n(%)		
Schizophrenia	29 (42)	21 (38)
Affective	19 (28)	14 (25.5)
Paranoid state	5 (7)	5 (9)
Neuroses	11 (16)	5 (9)
Alcoholism	3 (4)	3 (5.5)
Anorexia nervosa	0 (0)	1 (2)
No illness	2 (3)	6 (11)

BSO: behaviour and other syndromes; DAH: delusional and hallucinatory syndromes; NSN: non-specific neurotic syndromes; SNS: specific neurotic syndromes; PSE:
[a] Four people from each group refused to be interviewed.

the Sparkbrook group both at the initial assessment and at the 1 month assessment.

The relatives of Sparkbrook patients were more satisfied with the treatment and the support and help they themselves had received. This was probably due to the fact that the Sparkbrook patients had more face to face contacts with a psychiatric nurse than the Small Health group in the first month and at one year 56% of the patients were still in contact with a community nurse compared with only 14.5% of the Small Health group. More patients were also in contact with a psychiatrist at one year (81% versus 62%).

The characteristics of the people admitted from Sparkbrook during the study are of interest and may improve our understanding of who benefits from which kind of treatment. As one might expect the people who were admitted were more likely to be regarded as a danger to others although some were treated at home. People who were suicidal or had made a suicide attempt were infrequently admitted and only three (of 19) patients who were regarded as a suicide risk and two (of 14) people who had attempted suicide were admitted during the study. People who ived alone, were non-compliant with treatment and were young and nale were also more likely to be admitted.

Conclusion

The service provided in Sparkbrook is successful in keeping in contact with people with long-term disability and provides a service which they ike to use. The service is also well taken up by people from Asian and Caribbean cultures. It is preferred by relatives but is not suitable for everyone; around 30–40% of people still require admission. The social and symptomatic outcome is not different between the two groups. The next step is to define more clearly the characteristics of people who would benefit most from which package of care. The continual audit of the service is useful to this end and it also facilitates flexibility of the service in response to the changing needs of the population.

References

Dean C, Gadd EM (1990). Home treatment for acute psychiatric illness. *British Medical Journal*, **301**: 1021–3.
Dean C, Phillips J, Gadd EM *et al.* (1993). A comprehensive community based service for people with acute severe episodes of illness. *British Medical Journal* **307**: 473–6.
Grad J, Sainsbury P (1968). The effects that patients have on their families in a community care and a control psychiatric service – a two year follow-up. *British Journal of Psychiatry*, **114**: 265–78.
Hoult J, Reynolds I (1985). Schizophrenia: a comparative trial of community oriented and hospital orientated psychiatric care. *Acta Psychiatrica Scandinavica*, **69**, 359–72.
Jarman B (1983). Identification of underprivileged areas. *British Medical Journal*, **286**: 1705–9.
Patmore C, Weaver T (1991). *Community Mental Health Teams: Lessons for Planners and Managers*. Good Practices in Mental Health, London.
Patmore C, Weaver T (1992). Improving community services for serious mental disorders. *Journal of Mental Health*, **1**: 107–15.

5

Early intervention study of psychiatric emergencies

PETER TYRER

Introduction

Although the randomised controlled trial is still the best available method of comparing different service strategies as well as its more conventional role in the evaluation of treatment, there are many problems preventing generalisation from the findings. To some extent it is always artificial to compare 'hospital' and 'community' services because in practice all hospital services have some community elements and few community services, if they are truly comprehensive, have no hospital components. Another important methodological problem is that from the initial pioneering studies of Stein & Test (1980) onwards, most of the community services being tested have been set up as a consequence of a research programme and can therefore in no way be regarded as part of a standard service. The findings of such studies, although of great interest, may have no bearing on services in other parts of the country where similar resources are not available. Research teams who are highly motivated, often spurred as much by the academic questions associated with their research as in commitment to their day to day service, are in no way representative of services as a whole.

The issue of burn-out, which has often been attributed to community teams (Dedman, 1993), also cannot be addressed adequately in studies that involve teams that have been especially introduced for the purposes of the research. If teams with a special interest in research are involved in setting up a service it is not surprising if their members move on when the initial flush of research activity ceases. This is not necessarily burn-out but clearly it is inappropriate for a team with a primary clinical function to have repeated changes in membership and direction.

The studies from Birmingham and Nottingham described in this book are more representative of what happens in practice because they describe established services developed for specific populations. These do not use the methodology of the randomised controlled trial. In our study of early intervention in psychiatric emergencies presenting in the Paddington area of London, we employed the randomised controlled trial to compare two existing parallel services and, to our knowledge, this is the first study to use this methodology without altering the existing service configurations.

We were able to do this because the community and hospital services in Paddington operated in parallel and yet were distinct. The community service (Early Intervention Service) was quite independent of the hospital (Standard) service yet there was considerable overlap in the populations treated. This is somewhat unusual because most community services that are independent of the hospital do not cater for the same populations and therefore cannot be compared in a randomised controlled study. To understand how the two services were operating in parallel in Paddington it is necessary to give more background information.

History of the Early Intervention Service

In 1987 the Early Intervention Service (EIS) was set up as a National Health Service (NHS) demonstration project in the London borough of Paddington and North Kensington. This borough has a population of around 120 000 (although it has many additional transient residents that are never counted in census figures). It contains many ethnic minorities and also many temporary residents, often from other London boroughs placed in hotel accommodation in the Paddington area. These factors, together with its inner city location, made Paddington and north Kensington the ninth most socially deprived area in London using the Jarman indices (Jarman, 1983). Many of the admissions to hospital in such areas are of patients with very serious mental illness. The EIS was specifically set up with the task of providing for the care of the severely mentally ill and although it operates an open referral system, severe mental illness always took priority. Although general practitioners are the most frequent referrers (35% of total) (Marriott *et al.*, 1993), evaluation of the cases referred showed that they generally referred less severe illness than other agencies. Similar findings were shown when all non-medical referrals were compared with others (Marriott *et al.*, 1993).

The service operates a policy of rapid response but is not a crisis intervention service and does not have 24-hour cover. It comprises a multi-disciplinary team of eight, including two community mental health nurses, two social workers, a psychiatrist, an occupational therapist, a psychologist and an administrator, with sessional help from junior psychiatrists. Most initial assessments are carried out in patients' homes and special attention is paid to special multi-disciplinary working, regular reviews and close liaison with other mental health agencies. The team from its beginnings in 1987 operated a case management system (Onyett, 1992) which is very similar to the care programme approach introduced by the Department of Health (DOH) (1990) in which each key worker takes major responsibility for patients under his or her care. The diagnostic and management decisions are reached by consensus at regular team meetings (Onyett *et al.*, 1990).

Approximately one in six of all referrals comprise emergencies presenting either directly to the local psychiatric unit (the Paterson Wing, St Mary's Hospital), the Accident and Emergency Department at St Mary's Hospital or to the duty psychiatric social worker. It was felt that this population would be the most appropriate to evaluate in a randomised controlled trial because patients presenting to those setting could be referred equally to the Standard service or the EIS under normal clinical circumstances.

Study design

Patients presenting as emergencies to the psychiatric service at St Mary's Hospital, Paddington, in a 14-month period (May 1989 to June 1990 inclusive) were considered for the study if they were aged between 16 and 65 years, judged after assessment by the psychiatrist or approved social worker to be suffering from a psychiatric disorder other than primary alcohol or drug dependence, were resident within Paddington, did not require mandatory inpatient psychiatric care, were not in current contact with the psychiatric services and gave informed consent for the study.

Patients meeting these criteria were immediately allocated to the EIS or Standard (control) groups by the duty psychiatrist or approved social worker opening a sealed envelope giving random allocation. Patients were stratified for the presence or absence of previous psychiatric contact as this was considered an important prognostic variable.

Patients randomised to two services received the normal treatment in that service and no changes were made that might have interfered with normal practice. The choice of treatment in both services was determined entirely by clinicians with no restrictions imposed by the study design. In practice most EIS referrals were seen at home initially and Standard referrals seen in psychiatric outpatient clinics with occasional domiciliary visits by senior psychiatrists.

At original randomisation patients were referred for research assessment by a psychiatrist blind to service allocation. Psychiatric symptoms and signs were scored using the Comprehensive Psychopathological Rating Scale (CPRS) (Åsberg *et al.*, 1978) and its subscales for depression (Montgomery & Åsberg, 1979) and anxiety (Tyrer *et al.*, 1984). Social function was measured using the Social Function Questionnaire (SFQ) (Tyrer, 1990), a self-rated eight-item questionnaire which correlates highly with the Social Function Schedule, an observer-rated instrument (Remington & Tyrer, 1979; Tyrer *et al.*, 1990).

Further assessment and scoring of CPRS and SFQ were carried out 2, 4 and 12 weeks after randomisation, either at home or hospital depending on patients' preference. Efforts were made to maintain the research interviewers' ignorance of service allocation; if this information were revealed later interviews were carried out by a second psychiatrist blind to this knowledge.

Results

These have been reported in full elsewhere (Tyrer, 1992; Merson *et al.*, 1992; Tyrer *et al.*, 1994) and are only briefly presented here. Two major findings that are consistent in most comparisons of community and hospital services were that the bed occupancy was significantly less in patients referred to the EIS and this was particularly marked for patients with schizophrenic diagnoses (Tyrer, 1992) (Figure 5.1). The second finding consistent with other studies was the much greater satisfaction with services in patients treated by the EIS compared with the Standard service. This was accompanied by a much higher rate of successful contact with patients in the community service, so that only one of the 48 patients in the community service was not seen compared with 15 of 52 in those randomised to the hospital service. There was also a greater range of treatments given in the EIS whereas most treatment in the Standard service consisted of psychotropic drugs (Merson *et al.*, 1992).

Patients referred to the EIS also showed somewhat greater improvement in psychiatric symptomology over the 12 weeks of the study. This

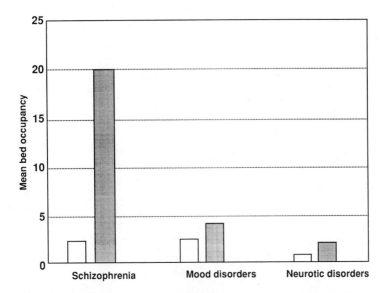

Figure 5.1 Mean duration of bed occupancy in patients randomised to the community service (EIS) and standard hospital service with schizophrenia (*n* = 19 for EIS and Standard), mood disorder (*n* = 12 (EIS) and *n* = 20 (Standard)) and neurotic disorder (*n* = 13 (EIS) and *n* = 12 (Standard)). Four patients were found to have a substance abuse disorder after initial assessment but none was admitted to hospital. (■) Standard. (□) EIS.

was most marked for total scores on the CPRS for the 85 patients who completed the study (Figure 5.2) but was less marked when re-analysis, taking into account missing data, was carried out (Merson *et al.*, 1992).

Implications of the findings in conjunction with those of other studies

The findings that patients prefer community treatment and occupy fewer psychiatric beds are consistent with the other studies reported in this volume and suggest that even though the population being seen was less ill than those involved in care at the point of inpatient treatment the same principles apply. The relatively small but significant difference in clinical outcome is also similar to the findings of some studies (e.g. Hoult & Reynolds, 1985) and shows clearly that patients were not disadvantaged by having shorter periods in hospital.

It is also possible to argue that it is easier to generalise in these findings than those of other published studies because this study involved two

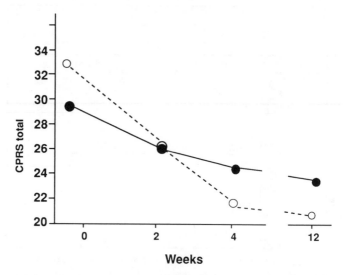

Figure 5.2. Mean improvement in total psychopathology on the Comprehensive Psychopathological Rating Scale (CPRS) in 85 patients presenting as emergencies and randomly allocated to the Early Intervention Service (EIS, --○--) and the hospital based service (Standard, —●—). F-ration (service/time interaction) = 3.39; d.f. = 3, 249; P = 0.019.

services working in parallel. There are several criticisms, however, that need to be answered before such generalisation can be made. Firstly, the selection of the patients in the study clearly excluded a large number of patients who present to psychiatric care and are often admitted to hospital. By excluding patients who needed mandatory admission (those under compulsory orders and those for whom such orders might have been made if voluntary admission was not agreed) it is quite possible to argue that the EIS was only effective in a select group of patients who were not representative of the population as a whole. This argument has some merit although it is important to emphasise that psychiatric emergencies constitute the most frequent root of admission to hospital and that those seen in the study included many who were not considered for admission by either service and would therefore tend to dilute the findings. If we had extended the entry criteria of the study to include all patients presenting to the services, the EIS would not have been operating in its normal 'mode' and therefore the criticisms mentioned at the beginning of this chapter would have applied to the study.

The second criticism is that the study only took place over a period of 12 weeks and the findings may have been different over a longer period. Again this has some merit as a criticism but patients who present as psychiatric emergencies, particularly in an inner city area, often have limited residential status in the area and we would probably have lost contact with any more individuals if the study had been carried out over a longer period.

Lastly, the differences could be put down a greater motivation and enthusiasm of the community team and may therefore be a measure of these qualities rather than any intrinsic merit of the service strategy. This is always a difficult point to refute, not least because it is impossible to separate merit and enthusiasm from other variables. If the service is working well and with apparent efficiency, it is not surprising that those working in it have greater morale and are more enthusiastic than in other settings. The therapists in both services knew about the referrals and were aware of the independent assessments. The EIS is a clinically orientated team which dislikes interference in what it considers to be its essential work and the independent research involved in this study was not received enthusiastically, as to some extent it interfered with normal day to day clinical work (e.g. ensuring that patients did not disclose information about the service to the assessors, together with other measures such as arranging places of appointment differently in order to maintain masking of assessors' knowledge). During the 20-month period of the study, 252 new patients were seen for care by the service so that the 48 referred to the EIS only constituted 17% of the total. The research evaluation was therefore only a relatively small part of the total work of the team.

Taken together, it is reasonable to argue that the findings of other studies, particularly those concerning greater service satisfaction and reduction of in patient beds, are still shown when existing community and hospital services are compared. In other words, the results do not merely flow from specific research interest or increased resources. They also show that when a community team such as the EIS concentrates specifically on severe mental illness it has a positive impact on bed usage without any impairment in terms of pathology.

The nature of working relationships in the EIS, which preceded the care programme approach of the DoH, also suggests that when care programming operates intensively, with regular reviews (in the EIS all patients are reviewed every week) and this works well with high patient satisfaction, reduced use of in-patient facilities and favourable clinical outcomes. Independent evidence from other work of the EIS suggest that these conclusions can be reinforced and that the team also has a favourable impact on suicide rates.

Conclusion

This study shows that a community based service concentrating on the care of the severely mentally ill is effective in keeping patients out of hospital, improving satisfaction of patients with the service and is more effective than the equivalent hospital service in reducing psychopathology. It is also relatively cheap. How much of the success of the service depends on the individual personalities within the team (who have remained remarkably constant over the 6 years that the service has been functioning) and how much is related to the operational function of the team is not possible to evaluate but should become clear as similar models of care are tested and compared.

References

Åsberg M, Montgomery SA, Perris C, Schalling D, Sedvall G (1978). A comprehensive psychopathological rating scale. *Acta Psychiatrica Scandinavica*, Suppl. **271**: 5–29.

Dedman P (1993). Home treatment for acute psychiatric disorder. *British Medical Journal*, **306**: 1359–60.

Department of Health (1990). *Community Care in the Next Decade and Beyond*. HMSO, London.

Jarman B (1983). Identification of underprivileged areas. *British Medical Journal*, **286**: 1705–9.

Hoult J and Reynolds I (1985). Schizophrenia: a comparative trial of community oriented and hospital oriented psychiatric care. *Acta Psychiatrica Scandinavica*, **69**: 359–72.

Marriott S, Malone S, Onyett S, Tyrer P (1993). The consequences of an open referral system to a community mental health service. *Acta Psychiatrica Scandinavica*, **88**: 93–7.

Merson S, Tyrer P, Onyett S, Lynch S, Lack S, Johnson AL (1992). Early intervention in psychiatric emergencies: a controlled clinical trial. *Lancet*, **339**: 1311–14.

Montgomery SA, Åsberg M (1979). A new depression scale designed to be sensitive to change. *British Journal of Psychiatry*, **134**: 382–9.

Onyett S (1992). *Case Management in Mental Health*. Chapman and Hall, London.

Onyett S, Tyrer P, Connolly J *et al.* (1990). The Early Intervention Service: the first eighteen months of an Inner London demonstration project. *Psychiatric Bulletin*, **14**, 267–9.

Remington M, Tyrer P (1979). The Social Functioning Schedule: a brief semi-structured interview. *Social Psychiatry*, **14**: 151–7.

Stein LJ, Test MA (1980). Alternative to mental hospital treatment. 1. Conceptual model, treatment program and clinical evaluation. *Archives of General Psychiatry*, **37**: 392–97.

Tyrer P (1990). Personality disorder and social functioning. In: Peck DF, Shapiro CM (eds) *Measuring Human Problems: a Practical Guide*, pp. 119–42. John Wiley, Chichester.

Tyrer P (1992). Schizophrenia: early detection, early intervention. In: Jenkins R, Field V, Young R (eds) *The Primary Care of Schizophrenia*, pp. 51–7, HMSO, London.

Tyrer P, Owen RT, Cicchetti D (1984). The Brief Scale for Anxiety: a subdivision of the Comprehensive Psychopathological Rating Scale. *Journal of Neurology, Neurosurgery and Psychiatry*, **47**: 970–5.

Tyrer P, Merson S, Harrison-Read P, Lynch S, Birkett P, Onyett S (1990). A pilot study of the effects of early intervention on clinical symptoms and social functioning in psychiatric emergencies. *Irish Journal of Psychological Medicine*, **7**: 132–4.

Tyrer P, Merson S, Onyett S, Johnson T (1994). The effect of personality disorder on clinical outcome, social networks and adjustment: a controlled trial of psychiatric emergencies. *Psychological Medicine* (in press).

6

Evaluation of psychiatric services: the merits of regular review

BRIAN FERGUSON

Introduction

Nottingham has followed an evolutionary path in the development of community psychiatric services. The present structure was heralded by innovations introduced during the 1950s and 1960s by Dr Duncan Macmillan, who was then superintendent of Mapperley Hospital. He began the process of discharging large numbers of long-stay patients who were living in the hospital by placing them in residential homes throughout various parts of the city. The unlocking of all wards areas in 1958 resulted in the acute admission services adapting their way of working to patterns which later facilitated the present concepts of community psychiatry (MacMillan, 1963).

The outward movement of patients led to the development of day facilities which initially functioned as Occupational Therapy departments for the long-term mentally ill. In time, acute day hospitals developed and began to take over some of the functions previously undertaken by acute wards. The first dedicated community Mental Health Centre was opened in the early 1980s and subsequently there has been a gradual extension of these services to all areas of the city.

Present services

The mental health needs of the City of Nottingham are to a large extent provided by the mental health unit, with limited private practice facilities. The district covers a population of areas in a wedge-shaped fashion so that each contains a part of the inner city. The catchment areas or sectors are served by a mental health team which has a community base from which the local psychiatric service is organised. Each of these bases has access to acute day hospital facilities and three of the northern sectors have day hospitals located on the community base site. The mental health teams are multi-disciplinary in nature and include social work, community psychiatric nurses, occupational therapists, psychologist and psychiatrists. Each sector has access to a 20-bed admission unit. For the southern sectors, this is located at Queen's Medical Centre and at the present time the admission facility for the northern sectors is located at Mapperley Hospital, which is designated to close shortly. In addition, there are district-wide specialist services, which include Drug and Alcohol, Health Care of the Elderly, Psychotherapy, Rehabilitation and Child and Adolescent Psychiatry.

Evaluation of psychiatric services

The present services in Nottingham have gradually evolved over a 25-year period. Innovations such as the introduction of community-based mental health teams and liaison clinics in general practice have generally been forged in one or other of the sectors before becoming an accepted model of practice. Once they have been up and running, and have shown their value, they have been introduced by the other sector teams. This evolutionary path has proved beneficial in that it has allowed comparative evaluation which would otherwise not be possible.

In its search for methods to assess the benefits and disadvantages of service changes, Nottingham has not followed the model of randomised controlled trials. Although such techniques can effectively evaluate a particular component of service, they cannot adequately mimic the reality of clinical practice, once services are up and running. Randomisation, for example, removes the very important components of clinical decision-making that may determine the perspective of a given service, especially in such sensitive areas as patient selection for therapy. The other difficulty which can arise is that the component chosen for evaluation may bear no true relationship to what can be made routinely available in clinical practice and therefore the results of the comparison may not be generalisable to other services.

The changes in Nottingham occurred on a staggered basis, because of which it has proved possible to compare services which represent radically different approaches. A previously published study (Ferguson *et al.*, 1992) used the technique of comparing two cohorts of patients who had received treatment in either a hospital or community orientated service over a protracted period. The Nottingham Case Register was used to identify two comparable groups, matched for age and sex in addition to level of care, which had received treatment during the index year 1983. Their progress during a subsequent 5-year period was recorded and they were then visited in their homes by a research assistant, who conducted an assessment of mental state, social functioning and satisfaction from both the patient's and carer's points of view.

Mental state was assessed using the Comprehensive Psychopathological Rating Scale (CPRS) (Montgomery & Åsberg, 1989) and the patients' perception of their level of social functioning evaluated by means of the Social Functioning Schedule (SFS) (Remington & Tyrer, 1979). The results (Table 6.1) indicated that there were no statistically significant differences between the two groups on either of these parameters. The community services, however, appeared to be effective in delivering a similar quality of care to an area of very high social disadvantage, as determined by Nottingham County Council deprivation data (Nottingham County Council, 1983). At the 5-year follow-up stage, there was also a higher proportion of patients still in care within the community service compared with the hospital group (33% versus 6%), with greater input from senior medical staff who remained involved in their treatment (83% versus 57%).

One of the difficulties in this approach is that although it can provide a longitudinal view of service delivery it tends to yield only cross-sectional views of symptomatology. It is possible, as in the above example, to control for age and sex but there are still a great number of differences between such cohorts which can act as confounding factors. Clinical trial methodology with serial assessments may, paradoxically, also result in inaccurate evaluations because the assessments themselves may exert a significant impact on the service experienced by the patient. Service evaluations should therefore be multi-faceted so that symptom/social outcome measures are combined with other assessments.

Process data

The standard way of looking at psychiatric services has been to examine activity data, particularly in relation to hospital admissions. The presence of a well-established Case Register has allowed the Nottingham Service to take a balanced longitudinal view of the impact which community patterns of working exerted on admissions and a variety of other clinical contact rates in outpatient and day hospital settings. A number of studies have been published (Tyrer *et al.*, 1984, 1990) and have shown, for example, a reduction in admission rates of 30% between the years 1978

Table 6.1 *Evaluation of a community service*

	MADRS score	BAS score	Schizophrenia subscale score	Obsessional subscale score	Total CPRS score	SFS score
Community cohort						
Mean	4.19	6.45	2.08	2.88	15.13	20.70
95% CI	3.56–4.81	5.71–7.12	1.67–2.50	2.49–3.28	13.48–16.78	13.31–20.39
Hospital cohort						
Mean	4.46	6.28	2.0	3.18	14.59	22.68
95% CI	3.57–5.34	5.33–7.23	1.53–2.47	2.67–3.68	12.30–16.89	18.89–26.48
Removing the effects of social deprivation score as covariate						
Differences between adjusted means for hospital and community cohorts[a]	1.05	−0.76	−0.31	−0.70*	−2.20	1.54
Standard error	0.58	0.62	0.33	0.34	1.5	2.76

Means and 95% confidence intervals for symptom outcome measures.
BAS: Brief Scale for Anxiety; MADRS: Montgomery and Åsberg Repression Rating Scale
[a] A positive difference favours the hospital service, a negative difference favours the community service.
* $P < 0.01$.
Source: Ferguson *et al.* (1992).

Table 6.2 *Patients' view of Community Service obtained by
questionnaire (n = 279)*

10%	Preferred to be seen at a different location
92%	Felt that their therapist was helpful
32%	Waited more than 15 minutes for their appointment when seen by a psychiatrist
9%	Waited more than 15 minutes for their appointment when seen by a Community Psychiatrist Nurse
92%	Felt their therapist understood what they were saying

and 1985 when some of the community initiatives were introduced. The case register provided evidence for an increased referral rate and greater use of day care facilities. The collection of routine data on such a large scale allowed comparisons with national figures. For example, a local fall of 37.5% in the use of inpatient beds compared favourably with a 24.2% national reduction in the same period (Tyrer *et al.*, 1989).

Other methods of service assessment

Traditionally, service industries look to their customers to measure their effectiveness. In psychiatry, there are a broad number of consumers, including the patient, carers, society at large and other professional groups. Clinicians have, perhaps, been a little reluctant to ask outsiders to comment on their work. There has been a hesitancy in approaching psychiatric patients themselves, in view of what might be considered to be their problems of judgement arising from the nature of their illness. There is also a worry that they may be heavily biased in favour of positive responses in circumstances where they are potentially dependent on their therapist. Patient satisfaction surveys in Nottingham, however, have proved to be a valuable tool in that patients appear to be able to give an objective negative response when they disapprove of some aspects of the service received (Table 6.2). They have shown themselves willing to make individual critical comments, including those of a positive nature, and indeed this has led to a very strong advocacy movement emerging in Nottingham. To date, patient satisfaction surveys have proved most effective at providing general satisfaction measures but have been less good at distinguishing between the more subtle organisational aspects of service delivery.

One way around this dilemma has been to use a professional group to

Brian Ferguson

Table 6.3 *General practitioner satisfaction with four different local psychiatric services in the country of Nottinghamshire*

Service	No. of GPs surveyed	Very dissatisfied(%)	Dissatisfied(%)	Satisfied(%)	Very satisfied(%)
A	33	4	25	54	14
B	55	18	46	28	0
C	39	0	5	72	8
D	36	0	3	72	14

GPs: general practitioners.

evaluate the psychiatric service. General practitioners have participated in surveys of this nature for some time (Table 6.3). The Stirling County Studies (Leighton, 1982) have previously shown how effective they can be at picking up problems within psychiatric services, before the services themselves have become aware of what is happening. Although general practice may have a different agenda from psychiatry, it is possible to control for this in questionnaire design. Repeated evaluations several years apart can monitor the effectiveness of changes within a service and are particularly useful when combined with other measures.

Summary

The approach towards evaluating psychiatric services in Nottingham has departed from randomised comparisons, partly because these may lead to distortion and fail to reflect the true quality of the service when it is in operation over a longer period. Matched cohorts which have experienced particular styles of services have been compared and a number of other methods are used, including surveys of patients, carers and general practitioners. In essence, this approach parallels the conduct of a Ministry of Transport (MOT) vehicle test after the car has been up and running for a while. It obviously contrasts with the more scientific testing of individual components in laboratory conditions which is potentially similar to what is achievable in a randomised controlled trial. The MOT approach, however, can be appropriately standardised and can tell considerably more about the health of the vehicle well after it has approached operational maturity, as well as emphasising the important component of monitoring function at regular intervals.

References

Ferguson B, Cooper S, Brothwell J, Markantonakis A, Tyrer P (1992). The clinical evaluation of a new Community Psychiatric Service based on general practice psychiatric clinics. *British Journal of Psychiatry*, **160**: 493–7.

Leighton A (1982). *Caring for Mentally Ill People: Psychological and Social Barriers in Historical Context.* Cambridge University Press, Cambridge.

MacMillan D (1963). Recent developments in community mental health. *Lancet*, **i**: 567–71.

Montgomery S, Asberg M (1979). A new depression scale designed to be sensitive to change. *British Journal of Psychiatry*, **134**: 382–9.

Nottinghamshire County Council (1983). *Disadvantage in Nottingham, County Deprived Area Study*, Part 1. Nottingham County Council, UK.

Remington M, Tyrer P (1979). The social functioning schedule – a brief semi-structured interview. *Social Psychiatry*, **14**: 151–7.

Tyrer P, Ferguson B, Wadsworth J (1990). Liaison psychiatry in general practice – the comprehensive collaborative model. *Acta Psychiatrica Scandinavica*, **81**: 359–63.

Tyrer P, Seivewright N, Wollerton S (1984). General practice psychiatric clinics: impact on psychiatric services. *British Journal of Psychiatry*, **143**: 15–19.

Tyrer P, Turner R, Johnson AL (1989). Integrated hospital and community psychiatric services and use of inpatient beds. *British Medical Journal*, **299**: 298–300.

7

A home based assessment study

TOM BURNS

Introduction

A number of outreach services providing comprehensive specialist psychiatric assessment and care have been evaluated (e.g. Fenton *et al.*, 1979; Stein & Test, 1980; Dean & Gadd, 1990). All achieved significant reductions in inpatient care and none of these 'alternatives to hospitalisation' studies found the hospital based service superior (Braun *et al.*, 1981). The improved clinical outcome and consumer satisfaction with a possible cost saving demonstrated in Madison (Weisbrod *et al.*, 1980; Stein & Test, 1980) has stimulated a number of replication studies of their 'Training in Community Living' approach (Hoult *et al.*, 1983; Muijen *et al.*, 1992).

Despite their consistency, these findings are slow to translate into policy. In the UK, reservations about their generalisability to local conditions persist. Firstly, British sector services must meet virtually all the mental health needs of their defined populations and some patient groups might not respond to experimental approach or perhaps suffer relative therapeutic neglect (Stefansson & Culberg, 1986). Secondly, study staffing levels are much higher than is customary here. Stein and Test documented a rapid loss of their gains after special funding was withdrawn (as did Langley *et al.* (1969) and Davis *et al.* (1972)). Thirdly, neither Stein and Test's nor Hoult's control services offered continuity of inpatient and outpatient care or any significant contribution from primary care services. Lastly, how much is due to novelty and the investigator's zeal? Were the experimental services based on work practices and levels of motivation that are compatible with durable service provision?

The present study was designed to try and reduce these four biases.

The structure is a prospective controlled trial with patients randomly allocated either to an experimental or control service. Patients were assessed by a graduate researcher using semi-structured interviews within 2 weeks of clinical assessment and at 6 weeks, 6 months and 12 months. Available informants were interviewed at each point. Detailed records were kept of all service use.

Randomisation was at the point of referral so as to ensure a full range of disorders. Local sector teams with closely similar manpower were recruited in pairs to ensure equal resources and a fair balance of commitment to experimental and control services. Control services had well established multi-disciplinary working practices (Paykel *et al.*, 1982) and high quality staff.

One hundred and seventy-two patients entered the study over a 1 year period: 94 experimental and 78 controls. There were no differences in clinical outcome or social functioning. Treatment differences demonstrated a reduction in the proportion of patients admitted, the duration of admission and overall bed usage. This resulted in significant cost savings even when controlled for the imbalance between psychotic patients and non-psychotic patients in the two groups. The cost advantage to the experimental service falls below conventional levels of significance if tertiary specialist care is added but is increased if alcohol and brain damaged patients are excluded (Burns *et al.*, 1993*a,b*).

The services studied

The Dingleton Hospital model (Jones, 1987) was selected for study because of its proven durability over 30 years. This model proved acceptable to local consultants because of its durability but also because it stressed what was offered to patients (i.e. multi-disciplinary outreach) rather than what was to be avoided (i.e. hospital admission). The experimental teams agreed to assessments which were:

(1) Home based
(2) Joint (psychiatrist and other mental health professional)
(3) Within 2 weeks of referral.

There were no other limitations on the team's clinical decisions.

Detailed reports of the study and its findings have been published elsewhere (Burns, 1990; Burns *et al.*, 1993*a,b*). This chapter will focus on Team Structure and Staffing, Case Mix, those aspects of the study which distinguish it from others in the field, its most provocative findings and a discussion of its sustainability and generalisability.

Team structure and resources

Six Catchment Area Mental Health Teams were recruited to the study without strengthening of resources. Two teams served a more deprived inner city area (Wandsworth/Battersea) and four served more stable suburban areas (Mitcham and Wimbledon). Four consultants had split duties (special responsibility for rehabilitation, liaison, deaf unit) and contributed part-time to proportionately reduced catchment areas. All the teams operated in a multi-disciplinary manner and minor variations in staffing favoured neither group in any consistent manner.

Medical input was roughly equivalent to one full-time consultant and one full-time junior doctor per 40 000 population. Senior registrar input was small and variable. Each team had one full-time Community Psychiatric Nurse (CPN). These teams also had provision for a half-time joint appointment social worker and a half-time clinical psychologist. Not all of the psychology posts were filled. Since the study, the allocation of CPNs per team has increased to 1.5–2 WTEs (whole-time equivalents). There were no designated community occupational therapists or community mental health workers during the study period.

Bed allocation was equal between the services and varied between 0.2 and 0.3 acute beds per 1000 population with a degree of flexibility. Teams were responsible for their own inpatients with an identified inpatient nurse team on a shared ward. All apart from one team had their inpatient beds and day places located at Springfield Hospital.

No team had a community base at the time of the study. The community orientated teams operated out of ad hoc structures which included adding the community round on to the end of inpatients ward rounds, using the outpatient clinic secretary to administer the whole team and often drawing substantially on administrative input from CPNs. Lack of administrative structure was an extra burden on community teams during the study.

There is a long established tradition of multi-disciplinary working within the St George's Mental Health Unit. CPNs, psychologists and social workers are fully integrated into the Secondary Mental Health Team with few direct referrals. Most patients were referred by general practitioners to the team directly or to the team using the consultant's name. Half of the CPNs had been on English Nursing Board (ENB)

Table 7.1 *Initial patient characteristics*

Variable	Experimental $n = 94$	Control $n = 78$
Age: mean (years)	39	42
Male (%)	45	42
Married (%)	39	36
Living alone (%)	22	22
Owner occupier (%)	54	41
Employed (%)	35	28
Reg. Gen. Class: I and II (%)	15	15
Nationality: British (%)	79	77
Ethnicity: White (%)	94	88
Previous Psychiatric history (%)	46	44
Urgent referral (%)	12	20
Compulsory admission (%)	3	6
PSE catego psychotic (%)	29	43*
Median PSE total score at intake	15.5	16.5
PSE Case (5 +) at intake (%)	77	79

PSE: Present State Examination; Reg.Gen.: Registrar General.
*$\chi^2 = 6.75$, $P = 0.032$

CPN courses. None of the teams had any specific training for community work, and only one had previous experience of this way of working.

Patient characteristics

There was no targeting of patients in this study. All referrals were accepted unless found to be:

(1) In contact within the past 12 months
(2) Outside the age range in use by local clinicians (18–74 years)
(3) Outside the catchment area.

There were no exclusion criteria based on diagnosis, mode of referral or dangerousness. The range of patients accurately reflects that normally served by urban/suburban catchment area teams. The case mix, however, has an under-representation of the severely mentally ill. Table 7.1 shows the patients initial characteristics.

How this study differs

Firstly, this study examines services which were not run by 'product champions'. Only one of the three experimental teams had experience of, and commitment to, the model tested. The other two teams were interested but unconvinced. Impetus to engage in the trial arose partly from annoyance with over-simplistic criticism of psychiatric hospitalisation. The Hawthorne effect was therefore minimised. Given their modest commitment, the teams' compliance functioned as an ongoing measure of the face validity of the approach. In this it differed from previous studies where the experimental team was often specifically recruited with young, highly committed staff, benefiting from extra short-term rewards (PhDs, research publications, promotion, etc.).

Secondly, there were no extra resources. Experimental teams operated within normal manpower constraints and also lacked the necessary administrative structure for their work. If anything, therefore, there was a reduction in available manpower. No specific training was provided, so that extra skills were not available either.

Thirdly, the study also differed in having no clinical exclusion criteria. The impact on the whole range of patients could be studied and therefore more accurately reflect clinical reality. This would reduce the potential power of the study by including patients who are not benefited by the experimental approach. This was demonstrated (Burns *et al.*, 1993*b*) by a few brain damaged patients in the experimental group who substantially reduced its cost advantage.

Lastly, it should be stressed that the model tested was a very durable one, having proved itself sustainable over several decades in Scotland.

The most provocative findings

The most outstanding finding of this study is that a substantial and significant reduction in the need for inpatient care (and hence costs and disruption to patients' lives) can be achieved without extra resources by altering the style of assessment. Costs ranged from an excess of 40% to 70% for standard care, depending on how calculated (Burns *et al.*, 1993*b*). It is not clear which aspect of the changed assessment is responsible for the reduction in admission but undoubtedly both a reduction in admission rate and duration was achieved.

This would suggest that the advantages of integrated multi-disciplinary working are not being fully exploited at present within traditional team practices and that barriers towards more community based service can be lowered without the need for a massive transfusion of resources or skills.

Careful examination of the results suggests that the benefits of the

Tom Burns

Table 7.2 *Deaths during the study*

	Control	Experimental
Before psychiatric assessment	Natural	
	Suicide	
Before first research interview	Natural	
	Natural	
Before second research interview	Natural	Natural
Before third research interview	Suicide	Suicide
		Natural
Before fourth research interview	Suicide	

experimental approach are greater in the more deprived inner city sector with a higher concentration of psychotic patients. This reflects the findings of Stein and Test, and Hoult, who demonstrated much greater advantages to the experimental service than have been achieved here. Hospital admissions were reduced in psychotic patients but in non-psychotic patients few hospital admissions would be expected, leaving little scope for improvement. Concerns that excessive activity would be expended on less ill patients are not supported by this study. The average number of contacts per non-psychotic patient was no higher in the experimental group, although there was a suggestion that they occurred over a shorter period. The risk of the less severely ill patients monopolising precious specialist mental health care team time (Wooff *et al.*, 1988) may be reduced if non-medical and medical team members work closely together.

Failure to attend rates were substantially reduced from 20% to 7% by the experimental approach. There is no evidence from clinical intake profiles that this resulted in the 'sucking in' of patients with trivial disorders.

There was no evidence of an increased risk of suicide in our experimental group. Indeed, there was a suggestion of a reduced risk (Table 7.2). The fourth 'natural' control death was highly suspicious and probably suicide. Conclusions should not be drawn from such small numbers. One suicide occurred in the control group while the patient was awaiting assessment, there being no suggestion of urgency in the referral letter.

There is a suggestion from admission data that patients with no clear diagnoses were more likely to be admitted in the control services. The feasibility of going back for a second assessment interview and the availability of immediate support to patient and family while further

ssessment was conducted may reduce pressure on bed usage. We were
urprised to note that day hospital care was of marginal importance in
either service. Only 15 patients attended the day hospital during the
study and of those only five without going through an inpatient spell.

Is the service sustainable and generalisable?

The model tested has been used in rural settings in Scotland for 25 years
and it is, therefore, clearly sustainable with adequate resources. It has
operated for 8 years in a relatively settled suburban setting and since the
trial some aspects have been incorporated into local team policies. It has
not been tested over a long period in deprived inner city settings. The
results of this study, however, imply that its benefits are most marked
in these deprived areas. There are extra complications in very deprived
inner city areas with the risks to staff more often coming from the
neighbourhood through which they must pass rather than from the
patient. There is no evidence of increased staff burn-out or turnover
than from standard care in Dingleton or Wimbledon.

Major problems to its generalisability and sustainability may lie in
the expectations of professionals. There is resistance within the multi-
disciplinary team to the requirements for joint assessments. In particular,
clinical psychologists (and since that time some occupational therapists)
criticised it for encroaching on their professional independence. This
was particularly so with clinical psychologists who have realistic concerns
about the future of their discipline and need to document direct referrals.
In addition, some considered the arrangement to be 'infantilising'.
This objection was quickly overcome by experience of genuine shared
responsibility. Those who resisted most strongly may, however, be more
committed to their professional identity and be highly influential.

St George's Community Psychiatric Nurses are members of the multi-
disciplinary team and none is based in general practices. CPNs who are
used to direct referrals may be more resistant. Table 7.3 indicates the
substantially greater input from non-medical staff in experimental teams.
Resistance to joint assessment was rapidly eroded by experience and
may eventually be overcome with the resultant greater influence on the
clinical functioning of the team. Psychiatrists also are far from universally
positive about a more assertive community approach and there are a
number of obvious problems.

The consultant's time commitment to the team becomes transparent.
It is difficult to play a leading role in such a team without being

Table 7.3 *Distribution of outpatient/staff contacts*

	Control	Experimental
Consultant	179	125
Senior Registrar	37	67
Registrar/Senior House Officer	123	55
Total (%)	339 (75.7)	247 (47.9)
Community Psychiatric Nurse	91	202
Psychologist	15	49
Social Worker	3	18
Total (%)	109 (24.3)	269 (52.1)
Total	448	516

$P<0.001$, $\chi^2 = 77.6$.

available. Admitting patients to await a consultant's opinion becomes less acceptable. Team members rapidly develop high expectations of the medical members' involvement. This may conflict with other legitimate calls on consultant's time, such as serving on national committees, teaching, administration, etc.

Community psychiatrists are not contactable to colleagues for long periods so that brief but important telephone calls cannot be made or received between appointments, etc. This seriously complicates administrative obligations and is quite frustrating.

The work is less physically comfortable than office based practice. Traffic jams, climbing stairs and assessing patients in cold or dirty rooms is wearing. Unlike traditional domiciliary visits (DVs), these visits cannot be rushed in deference to the circumstances. They are the service cornerstone and must furnish a full and detailed assessment, both for clinical purposes and also to train juniors and medical students.

Community psychiatry seems less 'high tec'. The focus of the interview is inevitably broadened. This is often criticised by colleagues who insist that it is an inefficient use of time. While the results of this study suggest that it is not inefficient either in the teams' time or the patients' time what is reacted against is a lack of professional 'specialness'. Undoubtedly, the balance of outreach work emphasises the social more than the biological components in a comprehensive assessment. Doctors schooled in the pre-eminence of biological sciences need to regularly remind themselves of the value of social interventions and of this approach for their patients.

Multi-disciplinary community work may threaten the psychiatrist's status as a hospital specialist by emphasising similarities to general

ractice. This distancing from consultant colleagues by alternative work
ractices is compounded by geographical dispersal. This may have
mportant implications for the recruitment and training of future psy-
hiatrists. Many psychiatrists are concerned that the rapprochement
etween psychiatry and general medicine achieved during the past
0 years (significantly increasing the quality of psychiatric recruits)
ould be threatened by present developments. Multidisciplinary working
equires sustaining respectful relationships with colleagues from different
ackgrounds and highlights inevitable professional role conflicts. It is
lifficult to avoid them in this situation and solutions, although possible,
equire ongoing effort and commitment. Uni-disciplinary working within
nulti-disciplinary teams achieves conflict avoidance but perhaps at a cost
o the patient.

Lastly, consultants may feel understandably uncomfortable about
eing required to train junior doctors in ways of practising that are still
ovel to them. Certainly the first shared assessments can feel strange and
ut of control to clinicians with highly refined and long established work
outines.

Conclusions

There are a number of serious and legitimate concerns that need to
e addressed if effective community multi-disciplinary mental health
vorking is to be achieved. It is unlikely that any team member will will-
ngly abandon his/her professional specialness. However, the mounting
vidence (both at home and abroad) of the benefits to patients in terms
f less disruption and increased satisfaction, and to purchasers of a
nore cost-effective service, will ensure the spread of such practices. Our
tudy suggests that it is generalisable within the UK context and does
ot necessarily require extra resources to achieve significant benefits.
Having achieved such improvements and demonstrated a more goal
lirected efficient service, mental health professions should be able to
obby more effectively for adequate resources.

Acceptability of this multi-disciplinary approach may be hindered by
a failure to acknowledge that there are other, equally valuable, roles
or mental health professionals. Community psychiatry needs to see
tself as in cooperation with, not opposition to, academic psychiatry,
psychopharmacology, psychotherapy, etc. Not all psychiatrists (or nurses
or clinical psychologists for that matter) are temperamentally or ideo-
ogically suited to this sort of work. It is clearly sustainable by those who

82   *Tom Burns*

feel comfortable with it, as demonstrated in Dingleton or Wimbledon. It does, however, involve a continuous need to accommodate others' views and to compromise in a way that is not congenial to a substantial proportion of professionals. Its generalisability may be fostered better by recognising that it is one approach within public mental health provision and not the only one.

References

Braun P, Kochansky G, Shapiro R *et al.* (1981). Overview: deinstitutionalisation of psychiatric patients, a critical review of outcome studies. *America Journal of Psychiatry*, **138**: 736–7.

Burns T (1990), The evaluation of a home based treatment approach in acute psychiatry. In: DP Goldberg, D Tantam (eds) *Public Health and Social Psychiatry*, Hogrefe and Huber, Geneva.

Burns T, Raftery J, Beadsmoore A *et al.* (1993*a*). A controlled trial of home based acute psychiatric services. *I*. Clinical and social outcome. *British Journal of Psychiatry*, **163**: 49–54.

Burns T, Beadsmoore A, Bhat AV *et al.* (1993*b*). A controlled trial of home based acute psychiatric services. *II*. Treatment patterns and costs. *British Journal of Psychiatry*, **163**: 55–61.

Davis AE, Dinitz S, Pasamanick MO (1972). The prevention of hospitalisation in schizophrenics: five years after an experimental programme. *American Journal of Orthopsychiatry*, **3**: 375–88.

Dean C, Gadd EM (1990). Home treatment for acute psychiatric illness. *British Medical Journal*, **301**: 1021–3.

Fenton SR, Tessier L, Struening EL (1979). A comparative trial of home and hospital psychiatric care: one year follow-up. *Archives of General Psychiatry*, **36**: 1073–9.

Hoult J, Reynolds I, Powis MC, Weekes P, Briggs J (1983). Psychiatric hospital versus community treatment: the results of a randomised trial. *Australian and New Zealand Journal of Orthopsychiatry*, **17**: 160–7.

Jones D (1987). Community psychiatry in the Borders. In: Drucker (ed.) *Creating Community Mental Health Services in Scotland*, SAMH Publications, Edinburgh.

Langsley DG, Flomenhaft K, Machotka P (1969). Follow-up evaluations of family crisis therapy. *American Journal of Orthopsychiatry*, **39**: 753–9.

Muijen M, Marks IM, Connolly J, Audini B (1992). Home based care and standard hospital care for patients with severe mental illness: a randomised controlled trial. *British Medical Journal*, **304**: 749–54.

Paykel ES, Mangen SP, Griffith JH, Burns TP (1982). Community psychiatric nursing for neurotic patients – a controlled trial. *British Journal of Psychiatry*, **140**: 573–81.

Stefansson CG, Cullberg J (1986). Introducing community mental health services. *Acta Psychiatrica Scandinavica*, **74**: 368–78.

Stein LI, Test MA (1980). Alternative to mental hospital treatment. I. Conceptual model, treatment program and clinical evaluation. *Archives of General Psychiatry*, **37**: 392–7.

Weisbrod BA, Test MA, Stein LI (1980). Alternative to mental hospital.

II. Economic cost benefit analysis. *Archives of General Psychiatry*, **37**: 400–5.

Wooff K, Goldberg DP, Fryers T (1988). The practice of community psychiatric nursing and mental health social work in Salford: some implications for community care. *British Journal of Psychiatry*, **152**: 783–92.

8

Home treatment as an alternative to acute psychiatric inpatient admission: a discussion

FRANK HOLLOWAY

Introduction

Studies of home care as an alternative to inpatient treatment take place within the context of a long-term decline in psychiatric bed numbers, which began in the UK in 1955. Although much of this decline has been contributed to by the discharge and death of long-stay patients it has also been associated with a steady shortening of inpatient stays for 'acute' patients. Until the mid-1970s total admission rates increased, with a particularly dramatic increase in re-admissions. Subsequently admission rates have declined, a decline that has been more marked where sectorised services have been introduced (Tyrer et al., 1989). Psychiatric practice in the UK moved from the era of the locked mental hospital door via the 'open door' movement to the present revolving door of the District General Hospital psychiatric unit (Ramon, 1988).

More recently there has been a sustained effort to close the large psychiatric hospitals, replacing long-stay beds with local community provision and accommodation in private sector residential and nursing homes (Pickard et al., 1992; Leff, 1993). Carefully executed reprovision programmes do not result in an excessive rate of re-admission of former long-stay patients (Dayson et al., 1992; Pickard et al., 1992), although it is the heirs of this group (people with severe chronic and recurrent mental illnesses) who make the greatest demands on contemporary inpatient services.

It is interesting to speculate why these changes in bed utilisation have occurred. The initial impetus seems to have been changes in professional attitudes and practices within the psychiatric hospital rather than the implementation of government policy (Ramon, 1988). Although the psychotropic drug revolution undoubtedly contributed to the increase in patient turnover there have been few other obvious therapeutic advances in the intervening decades: certainly there is evidence that the quality of practical community support available to patients discharged after episodes of inpatient treatment for psychotic illnesses has not significantly improved in the past 30 years (Brown *et al.*, 1966; Melzer *et al.*, 1991).

Why the interest in home based treatment?

A number of factors have contributed to the current interest in home based care for people experiencing acute episodes of mental illness. Firstly, a small but influential body of studies from Canada (Fenton *et al.*, 1979), the USA (Stein & Test, 1980) and Australia (Hoult *et al.*, 1983) demonstrated the feasibility and (possibly) desirability of treating patients presenting for admission at home rather than in hospital. These studies were complemented by research into the use of day hospitals as an alternative to inpatient admission (Wilder *et al.*, 1966; Herz *et al.*, 1971) and the adoption of brief inpatient care policies, with or without transitional day and residential care (Herz *et al.*, 1977; Hirsch *et al.*, 1979; Gudeman *et al.*, 1985).

The attitudes of psychiatrists also changed. Hospital admission was no longer seen as the only response to psychiatric crisis. A small number of crisis intervention services were developed (Scott, 1980; Smout *et al.*, 1983; Waldron, 1983) which attempted to put into practice Caplan's theories (Caplan, 1961). Home treatment could also emerge as an option by building on existing Community Psychiatric Nursing Services, although this possibility was often vitiated by the activity of the Community Psychiatric Nurse (CPN) as an independent practitioner located within primary care rather than as a member of a multi-disciplinary psychiatric team. The improvement in general practitioner training in psychiatry may have allowed general practitioners to manage more episodes of illness at home, possibly with the advice and support of the consultant psychiatrist. (This aspect of practice receives surprisingly little attention in the primary care psychiatry literature.) The 1983 Mental Health Act put new responsibilities on the Approved Social Worker (ASW) to identify potential alternatives to compulsory admission prior to making an application under the Act. In practice, 'diversion' of referrals into alternative forms of care by ASWs are uncommon (Hatfield *et al.*, 1992) and to date the ASW role has not resulted in any significant development of community alternatives to admission by Social Service Authorities.

Two particularly powerful forces have further focused attention on alternatives to admission. Firstly, the rapidly rising costs of inpatient services at a time of severe financial restraint have led to significant bed closures as local managers of mental health services attempt to balance their budgets. These bed reductions, now overseen by Health Authority purchasers, are in line with local and national policies that perceive inpatient admission as by definition a bad thing and community care as naturally a good thing. Secondly, bed shortages, which are particularly acute in London (Hirsch *et al.*, 1992), have forced clinicians to adopt innovative approaches to managing their severely ill patients who cannot come into hospital.

Possible advantages of home based care

There are reasons to believe that home based care should have significant advantages over traditional hospital based care. With the 24-hour availability of a home treatment team the response to a psychiatric crisis might be more rapid than inflexible and inaccessible inpatient services. Treatment at home can make use of existing social and medical supports (family, friends, neighbours, the primary care team) in a manner denied to the inpatient unit. Home care may, arguably, be less stigmatising than inpatient psychiatric care, particularly when the local hospital has a bad reputation. (This problem will be of less relevance to people with severe disabilities consequent on a mental illness whose social conditions and behaviour already attract stigma.)

For patients with recurrent or chronic disorders treatment at home may minimise the negative effects of hospital admission. These include loss of social and instrumental skills and the development of dependence on services and institutional attitudes. Patients and carers may be empowered by the experience of managing an episode of illness without recourse to admission. In addition, specific treatments may be more appropriately carried out at home, for example family therapy and *in-vivo* skills training. Potentially, if the treatment has been carried out effectively and sensitively, a home based style of care may foster cooperation between the patient, carers and services. A trusted general practitioner or community nurse may be able to persuade an otherwise reluctant patient with a psychotic relapse to take medication. One often overlooked advantage of home based care is that follow-up and support of the patient and carers after resolution of the acute episode may be significantly better than that available within more traditional bed-oriented services (Melzer *et al.*, 1991). Finally and importantly in the current financial climate, home based care may turn out to be cheaper even if not clinically superior to traditional care.

Assessing studies of alternatives to admission

In an important paper reviewing the de-institutionalisation literature, Braun *et al.* (1981) spelt out methodological criteria for assessing studies of community alternatives to inpatient care. An adequate study should have 'internal validity', i.e. its conclusions should follow with a sufficient degree of certainty from the data presented. A study should also have 'external validity'. By this is meant 'what are the particularities with respect to such factors as case mix, institutional setting and other independent variables that are relevant as one considers generalising the results of credible studies into new programmes and policies'?

Braun *et al.* (1981) also identified a number of specific aspects of the design and conduct of a study that should be assessed.

There should be a clearcut method of allocation to the experimental or control condition (preferably random allocation).

Patients should be adequately characterised prior to randomisation using socio-demographic descriptors, psychiatric history, diagnostic data and psychosocial status.

There should be adequate description of experimental and control programmes, including the use of medication and other potentially important independent variables.

The outcomes of treatment should be measured by properly validated instruments with (if possible) observers blind to subjects' treatment allocation. (Outcome measures will include psychiatric symptoms and behavioural disturbance; social functioning; patients' social network and quality of life; the satisfaction of users and carers; carer burden; the occurrence of severely adverse events (such as suicide and homicide); and service utilisation and costs.)

Follow-up should cover a high percentage of cases and be for an adequate period.

Sample sizes should be adequate for appropriate statistical analyses. (Braun *et al.* (1981) particularly emphasise the dangers of a type II error where the sample size is inadequate.)

Research projects may involve a specially selected and committed staff group who work within the project over a limited time period. An important issue is therefore the sustainability of the service model adopted when it is applied over decades by staff of average competence and enthusiasm. It is also important to locate these studies within a broader epidemiological context and assess the impact of model programmes on the total mental health system (Bachrach, 1982).

UK studies of community alternatives to inpatient care

Two contemporary research projects involving the home care of people with acute mental illnesses have been carried out in the UK.

The Daily Living Programme

The Daily Living Programme (DLP) was designed as a replication of the work of Stein & Test (1980) and was carried out at the Maudsley Hospital which is located in a very deprived area of inner London. A descriptive account of the service (Marks *et al.*, 1988) and two reports of a controlled trial of home care versus standard treatment at the Maudsley Hospital have been published to date (Muijen *et al.*, 1992*a, b*). The study took in all new patients aged 18–64 years presenting for admission to the Maudsley Hospital via the Emergency Clinic from the surrounding catchment area and a 20% sample of re-admissions during a 25-month period. Patients were randomly allocated to 'standard hospital care' and to a home treatment condition, the DLP. Once engaged in treatment, the DLP continued to follow-up patients throughout the life of the study. The study included patients who were violent, suicidal and subject to compulsory detention under the Mental Health Act, although those with primary addiction or organic brain damage were excluded. The study population is therefore highly relevant to contemporary inner city psychiatric practice. An appropriate range of outcome measures was employed although the measure of social functioning that was used (the Social Adjustment Schedule (SAS); Weissman *et al.*, 1974) was not designed for use with a psychotic population: this could have resulted in a lack of sensitivity to change when applied to a socially handicapped group of patients.

There is evidence in the reported results (Muijen *et al.*, 1992*a*) of a possible problem in the randomisation procedure. Significantly more of the patients randomised to hospital care had previously been admitted to hospital ($\chi^2=5.4$, df=1, $P<0.02$). Studies of the decision to admit patients in an emergency room have found that admission is more likely to occur if the patient had been admitted previously (Marson *et al.*, 1988). It is therefore conceivable that in some cases at least Emergency Clinic staff interfered with the randomisation process by ensuring the admission of patients whom they knew and felt required hospital care.

It is important to note that the DLP did not prevent admission for 83% of the patients, although admissions were shortened very dramatically (Muijen *et al.*, 1992*b*). The DLP was also unable to prevent re-admissions, although again the total time spent by patients in hospital was very much less for those in the DLP.

In common with other home care studies (Stein & Test, 1980; Hoult *et al.*, 1983) there are a number of problems with the control condition, 'standard' care at the Maudsley Hospital. At the time of the study the criteria for admission to the Joint Hospitals may well have been unusual: certainly inpatient beds were more readily available than is the current experience in London. One of the most dramatic findings was an enormous reduction in bed days for DLP patients with neurotic illnesses: this must partly be an artefact of unusually prolonged admissions for control patients with neurotic diagnoses.

The 'pathways to care' of the study patients have not been discussed by the authors but are likely to have been 'deviant' in the sense of tending to be emergency presentations occurring without substantial involvement by general practitioners or recent prior contact with the services but often involving intervention by the police. These pathways to care are probably typical of inner city areas with poorly developed community services (Moodley & Perkins, 1991). The poverty of community services is also relevant to the outcome of patients at 18 months: by that time the study was in reality investigating the efficacy of good quality long-term community care versus inadequate community care rather than acute home care versus hospital care.

A number of further observations may be made. Firstly, the DLP proved the feasibility of offering home care for very severely ill patients within a highly socially deprived catchment area. The slight superiority in clinical outcome found at 18 months is, however, disappointing given the quality of the intervention offered by the DLP. The sustainability of the DLP approach, which was undoubtedly highly stressful on staff, is not proven since the project ceased taking on new cases after 2 years. The applicability of the DLP as a general approach to acute care within a catchment area has not been fully demonstrated as only a minority of all catchment area patients were included in the study.

It can be argued that the original project was based on a misunderstanding of the key lesson of Stein and Test's work, which in essence was not about providing acute care but about offering long-term assertive outreach for patients with severe mental illness. The focus on the acute episode, which tends to resolve whatever the treatment approach, obscures the importance of community support. Subsequent modification of the initial Madison service involved splitting responsibility for dealing with acute cases and long-term assertive outreach (Stein *et al.*, 1990).

The Sparkbrook service

The comprehensive community service for Sparkbrook, an inner city ward in Birmingham, has been in operation for a number of years (Dean & Gadd, 1989). The results of a study comparing Sparkbrook patients who were successfully managed at home with patients who were admitted to hospital has been published (Dean & Gadd, 1990). A subsequent study comparing the outcome for people from Sparkbrook experiencing acute episodes of psychiatric disorder with patients presenting for admission to a psychiatric service living in an adjacent catchment area has now been presented. It is worth emphasising that the home treatment programme at Sparkbrook is only one element of a much broader community service, which is based in a model community mental health centre.

The earlier descriptive study demonstrated that home treatment was feasible (Dean & Gadd, 1990) and the continuing existence of the service is a practical demonstration of its sustainability. The extent to which Sparkbrook is generalisable is not clear: certainly the tightly knit and supportive family structure of the very substantial local Asian population may have contributed to the success of the home treatment approach, which was carried out by a surprisingly small staff team.

The subsequent Sparkbrook study, which is still to be fully reported, is important methodologically because instead of a randomised controlled trial a comparative design was adopted. The randomised controlled trial, although the 'gold standard' of biomedical research, is most obviously applicable in deciding which of two or more specific treatments are more effective for a clearly identified clinical condition. The comparative approach is potentially able to identify the benefits (and problems) of broader service approaches: it could be argued that 'home treatment' of 'acute psychiatric disorder' is precisely the sort of problem that should be evaluated within a comparative design.

Observations on the home care literature

To date only five methodologically adequate contemporary studies of home care as an alternative to acute inpatient treatment have been carried out (in Montreal, Canada; Madison, Wisconsin; Sydney, Australia; South Southwark, London; and Sparkbrook, Birmingham). Given the importance of the issue and its implications for Mental Health Services the research base for a major shift towards home care is desperately thin and further studies are required.

Future controlled studies should have a firm epidemiological basis. The impact of a home care service on the total service system within a defined catchment area should be assessed. Comparisons should be made between home care and other current models of good practice, notably a well-integrated inpatient/community service, rather than with indifferent hospital oriented care. Studies should make use of the opportunities offered by natural experiments where sectorised services working in areas of similar socio-demographic characteristics adopt different service models.

The existing literature is significantly flawed in assuming that 'inpatient care' and 'home treatment' are specific treatments rather than locations for care: the 'black box' model of service provision predominates. In future studies both home care and control services should be characterised in detail: preferably there should be some form of training package associated with the innovative treatment.

The experience of receiving psychiatric care should be studied more thoroughly than the current trite 'user satisfaction' approach in order that therapeutic factors in both home care and inpatient care may be identified (Lieberman & Strauss, 1986). Very few studies have looked at what makes people better who are suffering acute episodes of psychiatric disorder. For example removal from a stressful environment, support from staff and fellow patients and drug treatment are obvious potential therapeutic factors for inpatient treatment. Some, but not all, of these elements are available to the person in receipt of home care. Future studies of home care also need to take account of recent therapeutic advances (for example the family management of schizophrenia, strategies to enhance the treatment compliance of psychotic patients and developments in cognitive-behavioural treatments).

One important but understated finding of the home treatment literature is the requirement for some residual inpatient service (Stein & Test, 1980). Inpatient units are likely to become increasingly difficult to manage effectively and to become more costly as the dependence of inpatients increases. Rising costs may offset some of the potential savings from home care services. The problems of inpatient wards may be compounded by difficulties that will be encountered in discharging patients with continuing disabilities who require supported residential care. In the UK access to scarce residential care will be further restricted following the implementation of the Government's community care reforms. Within the UK context it is also important that research is carried out on the impact of policy (particularly the application of the internal market and the community care reforms) on service provision. It is conceivable that policy will rebound against the development of effective community services. Purchasers may focus on 'core' bed based services and respond to central initiatives that appear to be demanding more not less inpatient provision, notably court diversion schemes and other initiatives to take the mentally abnormal offender out of the criminal justice system.

Successful home care services are likely to require additional resources in order to function effectively, for example readily accessed day care and crisis residential provision. These resources must be identified so that a comprehensive community oriented service can be properly costed. Researchers should be mindful of the fiscal crisis affecting health and welfare services. Cost-effectiveness, not to say cheapness, will be of the order of the day in the Mental Health Services of the next decade.

The development of unacceptable practices within hospitals dealing with the elderly, people with a mental handicap and the mentally ill has been well documented (Martin, 1984). Future research needs to focus on the training, support and supervision of staff working within home care services. Burn-out is potentially an important problem for stressed front line staff. Here the cynic might note that few of the people writing about home care actually practice it over a sustained period: we simply do not know if this style of work is feasible over a professional lifetime.

It would be tempting to read into the home care literature the lesson that hospitals are bad and community treatment is good. This is emphatically not the case, at least during the acute episode: there is no evidence that people initially improve more rapidly in non-hospital care. The outstanding lesson from the studies of home care published to date is that long-term assertive outreach and community support, focused on patients disabled by established severe mental illnesses is, to coin a phrase, the cornerstone of an effective psychiatric service.

References

Bachrach LL (1982), Assessment of outcome in community support systems: results, problems and limitations. *Schizophrenia Bulletin*, **8**: 39–51.
Braun P, Kochansky G, Shapiro R *et al*. (1981). Overview: deinstitutionalisation of psychiatric patients, a critical review of outcome studies. *American Journal of Psychiatry*, **138**: 736–49.
Brown GW, Bone M, Dalison B, Wing JK (1966). *Schizophrenia and Social Care*. Oxford University Press, London.
Caplan G (1961). *An Approach to Community Mental Health*. Grune and Stratton, New York.
Dayson D, Cook C, Thornicroft G (1992). The TAPS project 16: difficult to place, long-tem psychiatric patients: risk factors for failure to resettle long stay patients in community facilities. *British Medical Journal*, **305**: 993–5.
Dean C, Gadd E (1989). An inner city home treatment service for acute psychiatric patients. *Bulletin of the Royal College of Psychiatrists*, **13**: 667–9.
Dean C, Gadd E (1990). Home treatment for acute psychiatric illness. *British Medical Journal*, **301**: 1021–3.
Fenton FR, Tessier L, Streuning EL (1979). A comparative trial of home and hospital psychiatric care. One year follow-up. *Archives of General Psychiatry*, **36**: 1073–9.
Gudeman JE, Dickey B, Evans A *et al*. (1985). Four year assessment of a day hospital-in program as an alternative to inpatient hospitalization. *American Journal of Psychiatry*, **142**: 1330–3.
Hatfield B, Mohamad H, Huxley P (1992). The 1983 Mental Health Act in five local authorities: a study of the practice of approved social workers. *International Journal of Social Psychiatry*, **38**: 189–207.
Herz MI, Endicott J, Spitzer RL, Mesnikoff A (1971). Day versus inpatient hospitalization: a controlled study. *American Journal of Psychiatry*, **127**: 1371–82.
Herz MI, Endicott J, Spitzer RL (1977). Brief hospitalization: a two year follow-up. *American Journal of Psychiatry*, **134**: 502–7.
Hirsch SR, Craig T, Dean C *et al*. (1992). *Facilities and Services for the Mentally Ill with Persisting Disabilities*. Working Party Report on Behalf of the Executive Committee of the General Psychiatry Section of the Royal College of Psychiatrists.
Hirsch SR, Platt S, Knights S, Weyman A (1979). Shortening hospital stay for psychiatric care: effect on patients and their families. *British Medical Journal*, **1**, 442–6.
Hoult J, Reynolds I, Charbronneau-Powis M, Weekes P, Briggs J (1983). Psychiatric hospital versus community treatment: the results of a randomised trial. *Australia and New Zealand Journal of Psychiatry*, **17**: 160–7.
Leff J (ed.) (1993). The TAPS Project: evaluating community placement of long-stay psychiatric patients. *British Journal of Psychiatry*, **162** (Suppl. 19).

Lieberman PB, Strauss JS (1986). Brief psychiatric hospitalization: what are its effects? *American Journal of Psychiatry*, **143**: 1557–62.

Marks I, Connolly J, Muijen M (1988). The Maudsley Daily Living Programme: a controlled cost-effectiveness study of community based versus standard inpatient care of serious mental illness. *Bulletin of the Royal College of Psychiatrists*, **12**: 22–4.

Marson DC, McGovern MP, Pomp HC (1988). Psychiatric decision-making in the emergency room: a research overview. *American Journal of Psychiatry*, **145**: 918–25.

Martin JP (1984), *Hospitals in Trouble*. Blackwell, Oxford.

Melzer D, Hale S, Malik SJ, Hogman GA, and Wood S (1991). Community care for patients with schizophrenia one year after hospital discharge. *British Medical Journal*, **303**: 1023–6.

Moodley P, Perkins R (1991). Routes to psychiatric inpatient care in an inner London Borough. *Social Psychiatry and Psychiatric Epidemiology*, **26**: 47–51.

Muijen M, Marks IM, Connolly J, Audini B, McNamee G (1992*a*). The Daily Living Programme. Preliminary comparison of community versus hospital-based treatment for the seriously mentally ill facing emergency admission. *British Journal of Psychiatry*, **160**: 379–84.

Muijen M, Marks I, Connolly J, Audini B (1992*b*). Home based care and standard hospital care for patients with severe mental illness: a randomised controlled trial. *British Medical Journal*, **304**: 749–54.

Pickard L, Proudfoot R, Wolfson P *et al.* (1992). Mental Health Services in the Community. New Services in the Context of Hospital Closure. Evaluating the Closure of Cane Hill Hospital. *Final Report of the Cane Hill Research Team*. Research and Development in Psychiatry, London.

Ramon S (1988). Community care in Britain. In: Lavender A, Holloway F (eds) *Community Care in Practice*. John Wiley, Chichester.

Scott RD (1980). A family oriented psychiatric service to the London Borough of Barnet. *Health Trends*, **12**: 65–8.

Smout SM, Scott M, Fisher P (1983). Psychiatric crisis intervention in Tunbridge Wells. *Bulletin of the Royal College of Psychiatrists*, **5**: 46–8.

Stein LI, Diamond RJ, Factor RM (1990). A system approach to the care of persons with schizophrenia. In: Herz MI, Keith SJ, Docherty JP (eds) *Handbook of Schizophrenia*, vol. 5, *Psychosocial Therapies*. Elsevier, Amsterdam.

Stein LI, Test MA (1980). Alternative to mental hospital treatment. I, Conceptual model, treatment program and clinical evaluation. *Archives of General Psychiatry*, **37**: 392–7.

Tyrer P, Turner R, Johnson AL (1989). Integrating hospital and community psychiatry and reduced use of hospital beds. *British Medical Journal*, **299**, 298–300.

Waldron G (1983). Crisis intervention: is it effective? *British Journal of Hospital Medicine*, **31**: 283–7.

Weissmann MM, Klerman GL, Paykel ES, Prusoff B, Hanson B (1974). Treatment effects on social adjustment of depressed patients. *Archives of General Psychiatry*, **30**: 771–8.

Wilder J, Levin G, Zwerling I (1966). A two year follow-up evaluation of acute psychiatric patients treated in a day hospital. *American Journal of Psychiatry*, **122**: 1095–101.

9

The toxicity of community care

TIL WYKES

Introduction

This chapter is based, in part, on the overview of the studies (Chapter 1) and may will repeat some of the points made in Chapter 8 by Frank Holloway but perhaps in more detail. It will also focus on the possibility of generalising from these studies and whether the results can be sustained over time.

The run down of hospital based care was predicated on the positive effects for patients. In the community there are increased chances for continuing and practising skills as well as opportunities for widening patients' social networks. The process of case management offered in the community is also thought to encourage patients to take their medication and thus reduce levels of positive symptoms. The results of the experimental studies of novel community services discussed in this seminar, however, have all been disappointing.

Although I am not a 'product champion', I am one of the evangelists for community based treatments so you will understand how disappointed I am in the results. There have been no consistent positive findings except perhaps for greater user satisfaction with the services. Given that all the studies involved a committed, if not zealous, group of staff with reasonable resources these results put together are surprising. I would like you to bear in mind that I am a supporter of community care but I am nevertheless going to criticise the studies.

Why such poor results? The first step of any researcher who comes up with results contrary to expectations is to look at the design of the studies. Are there any features which would militate against finding positive results? For example would it have been possible to detect positive effects given the number of subjects, time for change and the

97

standard errors of the measures. I do not have access to the sort of data which would allow such detailed power analysis but it is clear that some measures will not change over the short periods of time encompassed by all the studies. For example some social roles, such as occupational or marital roles, are unlikely to change even over the 2-year period covered by the Daily Living Programme (DLP) project (Muijen *et al.*, 1992).

Is it possible to analyse the studies by amalgamating the data and thus increase the power of the tests? The assumption of homogeneity of the effects in each trial cannot be made because they are so different that a meta-analysis is not appropriate. It may be possible to divide up the degrees of freedom and test for individual effects in some sort of sensitivity analysis. For example the effect of community care can be examined for a particular diagnostic group or the effect of the particular treatments used in these trials. It may then be possible to make some comparisons because the variance between trials will have been reduced.

I am not going to dwell on the design features of previous studies because at this stage we need to look forward to new research. In fact, the search through the studies for a possible meta-analysis led me to some disturbing conclusions about the nature of the studies and treatments that have so far been tested. These personal views are mentioned in the sections below together with what I consider to be the specific design remedies for future studies. The first step in this process is to decide what constitutes community based treatments. The following deliberations are not comprehensive; I have chosen the elements I regard as crucial.

What makes up a community mental health service?

Although as suggested by Professor Creed in his opening remarks, a meta-analysis of the data from the current studies is not possible now, it may be a goal for the future. To do this we would need much more detail on community services to create a suitable data base. Table 9.1 shows the five main elements that I have chosen. The first element, mental health resources, is often described in papers on community psychiatric services but perhaps not in enough detail. Listing the personnel in a team does not indicate how much time they have available for patient oriented care and how much of their time must be spent in management tasks. We also need to know where is the site of treatment. In rural services it is likely to be users' homes. In inner city services it may be a mental health resource centre.

Most projects do characterise the patient population for which the

Table 9.1 *What makes up a community mental health service?*

Mental health resources
1. What is the multi-disciplinary team?
   nurses, doctors, social workers, clinical psychologists, counsellors, clerical support, trainee professionals
2. How much time is allocated for each professional?
3. What is the staff/patient ratio?
4. Treatment site?
5. Rehabilitation site?

Patients with mental health problems
1. Psychiatric diagnosis
2. Severity of social disability
3. Ethnic mix
4. Medication compliance
5. Exclusion criteria

Community resources
1. Housing arrangements
2. Transport availability
3. Geography: rural versus urban versus suburban
4. Socio-economic status of population
5. Family support available
6. Extent of mobilisation of community resources

Treatment approaches
1. Medication
2. Supportive therapy
3. Behaviour therapy
4. Analytic therapy
5. Skills teaching
6. Patient advocacy
7. Problem solving
8. Cognitive behaviour therapy
9. Psychological interventions for psychotic symptoms
10. Family therapies

Organisation of care
1. Case management approach
2. Key worker versus team
3. Assertive outreach
4. Size of service
5. Access to inpatient beds

service is responsible. Even when measures of social disability have been recorded they have been so coarse that they do not provide the necessary detail for comparison purposes. The measures are never likely to show changes over short periods of time because they do not reflect small changes in social status.

Community resources, especially following the implementation of the Community Care Act, will provide the background which supports community treatment. Areas where there are few resources allocated to hostel or group home care will provide different opportunities to those where these services are more available. Most published evaluative studies of community services in this country have been in urban or suburban areas. Those rural models that have been published in other countries (e.g. Santos *et al.*, 1993) have relied much more on family supports and infrequent visits. The family supports are present in some of the services discussed today (Dean & Gadd, 1990) but patients in many urban and inner city services have few family supports and the service may then require more mental health and other community resources to provide an equivalent level of care.

What is interesting about nearly all of the services described today is the lack of clear descriptions of the treatments offered to psychiatric patients. I have set out a number of options in Table 9.1 but it would not be possible to speculate how many of these treatments were provided in the evaluated community services. The distribution of personnel under the Mental Health Resources section will determine many of these treatments. For instance, if a psychologist is not present in the team then it is unlikely that psychological treatment for psychotic symptoms could be offered.

What treatment has been tested so far? All the services describe what they do as assertive outreach. But what is that? What is the nature of the therapeutic interaction that takes place in an acute day hospital or a patient's home rather than in a hospital ward. In fact by the brief descriptions provided, all that the services seem to be offering is the best of hospital care. By that I mean that when a patient comes into hospital he or she has a clinical assessment, they are given treatment (medication usually) and when they are a little better other services are called upon to sort out financial and social needs. Unfortunately, in some hospital services the care lapses between crises. What the community based models offer is good hospital care where there is continuous monitoring of problems to reduce crises and to prevent deterioration (as previously discussed in Chapter 8). The adoption of essentially similar treatments in different settings has meant that studies have only tested the effects of geography: dispersing the service into more accessible, less institutionalising places. It is hardly surprising then that community treatments show few differences from hospital based treatment. If this were a study in genetics the researcher would probably conclude that

Table 9.2 *What should a community psychiatric service do for patients?*

1. Reduce symptoms and distress
2. Improve social functioning
3. Case management outcome (reduce daily hassles and chronic difficulties)
4. Patients should be satisfied with the community service, more so than with other hospital based services

the effect of the genes (treatment approaches) far outweigh the effects of the environmental influences.

It is clear that the studies so far have tested the organisation of care rather than specific treatment. In fact, assertive outreach was supposed to improve compliance with medication but no study has produced data to evaluate even this treatment approach. What we need to know about the organisation of care is the need for a team approach or a key worker system. The Community Care Act will have some influence on the sorts of approaches adopted as one of its guidelines suggests that many of the tasks involved in social care should be carried out by different people.

Unfortunately there has been a confusion between treatments offered and the specific organisation of care in which that treatment is provided. The easiest example is giving medication either through a mental health resource centre, a hospital based clinic, a general practitioner health centre or through home visits by a Community Psychiatric Nurse (CPN). The effectiveness of the treatment will be based not only on the sort of medication offered but also the engagement of the user in therapy. This is one of the easiest examples although it has not been tested and would require a meta-analysis of many different services and studies.

What should a community psychiatric service do for patients?

As well as cataloguing the information required for a meta-analysis there is also a need to define what outcome measures are relevant for community care. Table 9.2 shows four categories of possible improvements that could be tested. This list is not comprehensive but again is a personal view of the key elements. Most studies measure symptoms but few ever consider the distress of the patient. The symptom measure often chosen is the Present State Examination (PSE) (Wing *et al.*, 1976). This measure was never designed to show symptom change but provides a detailed description of the symptom profile. The profile will change from an acute crisis to more stable states although, as with the coarse measures of social functioning, it is unlikely that any subtle changes in functioning will be reflected by this measure.

Social functioning measures are problematic. There is the difficulty of the slowness of change even in measures that are more fine grained, e.g. Social Behaviour Schedule (SBS) (Wykes & Sturt, 1986). In a recent 6 year longitudinal study of patients transferred to community services from Netherne hospital, (i.e. a chronic stable group) improvements in social functioning were only detected in those patients who had moved to more independent care for at least 3 years (T Wykes, 1994). None of the evaluative studies of community care discussed here covered this sort of period. Most of the studies ended at 1 year. Only the DLP project showed significantly more improvements in social functioning in the community than in the hospital service and these only appeared after 20 months. Not only are there problems in the time period for change but there are also problems in specifying what is good outcome, especially in the current economic climate. Researchers who designate financial independence for a group who are clearly unlikely to gain unsupported employment is a way of shooting themselves in the foot. It may be as useful to try to get people involved in satisfying hobbies and improving their daily living skills. This is particularly relevant in rural settings where the availability of transport as well as job vacancies will affect success in the job market.

Another indicator of outcome is the end result of case management. Although many studies specify this as a treatment its efficacy has only been tested as if it were part of the organisation of services. If case management has any function it is to reduce the levels of stress for their vulnerable clients. The stresses include daily hassles, life events and chronic difficulties. There are standard measures for these stresses, e.g. Daily Hassles Scale (Lazarus & Folkman, 1984) and the Life Events Scale (Brown, 1989) which could be adopted and which could act as covariates in the overall assessment of outcome. In other words, the excuse for less positive results would be the effect of increased stressors due to poverty, lack of social support or just inner city life.

Users need also to be satisfied with their services. This is likely to improve the use of such services and the take up of treatments. Although this seems to be one area where there are more positive results for community care, as Tom Burns has pointed out, the users of such community services probably thought they were getting a better service than those people allocated to hospital based care. In a service

Table 9.3 *The services should not be toxic*

Staff should not experience more: burn-out, distress, sickness, turnover, danger (violence from patients and from the public in carrying out the job)

Patients should not experience excess: mortality made up from risk of suicide and physical illness. There should also not be a higher risk of relapse (e.g. from living with High EE relatives)

Families should not experience more: financial problems, high burden, stress effects on ill health

The community should not experience increases in: community burden, e.g. on housing officers, general practitioners, the church, etc; violent and unpredictable behaviour (murder)

High EE: high expressed emotion

where all patients in a geographical area received the same care there was no differential level of satisfaction with those people who by virtue of their address received hospital based care.

Perhaps the evaluation of community care should not be determined simply by positive outcomes for the users especially as there have not been enormous signs of this happening. If users do prefer services to be based in the community perhaps this is a reasonable rationale for community based care. Our attention should now turn to making sure that services do not affect users adversely. In the following section I will try to describe what sorts of factors ought to be considered in this new approach.

Measuring the toxicity of services

Toxicity falls into four components: toxicity to staff, patients, families and the community. These are shown with some examples in Table 9.3.

Staff

The movement of services into the community affects the staff as well as the patients although little has been published on these effects. The effects on staff are particularly important in trying to answer the question of whether a particular service model is sustainable. Given the modest effects of community based treatments, a loss of morale and/or lack of qualified or experienced staff cannot provide the background service stability necessary for patients with recurring problems. This effect is likely to occur after the service has operated for a couple of years, when the spotlight of evaluation has been turned off.

The stress associated with community based treatments will involve increased responsibility, more face to face contact with patients, increased risks of violence from patients with less available support from other colleagues and an increased need for more therapeutic and welfare skills. Promotion prospects and staff development may be available only within a larger organisation such as a hospital. These factors are likely to lead to more staff turnover, more burn-out and higher sickness rates. Much of the strain produced by these factors may be offset by the increase in personal decision-making and control over the job structure, although this is still not clear. Many of the data are, however, not available from the research projects already discussed.

Staff problems are not only associated with new responsibility. The organisation of work may also affect staff effectiveness. For instance, visiting patients in their own homes without other colleagues has associated risks. Patients may live in high crime areas where there is a danger of mugging from other residents.

Patients

A recent study estimated the rate of suicide among psychiatric patients to be 50 times greater than in the general population (Fernando & Storm, 1984). It is for this reason that patients thought to be at risk are provided with a hospital bed so they can receive 24-hour care. Within community services this may not always be possible or thought to be appropriate. There is therefore still some risk of untoward incidents which not only includes suicide but also violence or threats of violence towards others. This is an area generally skirted around by proponents of community based services but it has to be clear:

(1) what is the risk
(2) whether this is higher than that experienced by hospital based services
(3) whether the risk in community services is acceptable in return for less institutionalised care.

Suicide rates in particular are difficult to assess because of problems in tracing unexpected deaths. There have, however, been two studies which have been published in 1992 which purport to test the effects of community care on suicide rates. The first was carried out on three UK Health

Districts where the numbers of suicides were small (Boer & Briscoe, 1992; Morgan, 1992). Both studies concluded that the suicide rate had not increased since the advent of community based treatments.

A more thorough analysis was carried out by Cantor (Cantor *et al.*, 1992) in Australia. He looked at the risk of suicide in the five Brisbane health districts over a 41-month period following the implementation of a comprehensive community care service. He found 34 suicides, a risk of 520 per 100 000. This is in comparison to 274 per 100 000 found in studies of inpatient services but is similar to another study of discharged patients carried out in Iowa where the rate was 611 per 100 000. In the Australian study, 94% of suicides were by people not attending the services, 345 were within 1 week of the last treatment and 59% within 3 months of entry to the community psychiatric services. Half the group were documented as being at risk. There were no particular factors which differentiated the group of completed suicides compared with a matched control group which is unlike previous hospital studies. Although there were no predictive factors it is clear that the first 3 months of entry to the community service are a particularly vulnerable period and at this time clients would benefit from some more intensive involvement.

Many of the suicides found by investigation in the Australian study were not documented in the case notes. The DLP group also found this to be the case when they investigated suicides in their control group who had been discharged from hospital. What is needed is a rigorous reporting system and/or specifically designed long-term prospective studies which collect data on suicide both those completed and the severe attempts within all community service models.

As well as the mortal risk of suicide there is also the problem of physical health. In a previous study of physical health problems in California, patients with mental health problems had physical illnesses which were not detected. One percent of these difficulties were thought to be causal factors in the mental illness; 45% of exacerbating diseases also had not been recognised (Koran *et al.*, 1989). Patients within community psychiatric services may not have frequent contact with medically quali- fied staff. Although hospital based care does not guarantee any more frequent contact with medical staff, the case for a lack of differential recognition of major physical disorders has not yet been made.

We do know that the risk of poor outcome is higher in groups of patients who live with a relative who is critical and/or over-involved with a patient (Kuipers, 1992). The effect of both community oriented services and the financial constraints now placed on supported housing decreases the chances of placements outside the family home. Dealing with the high expressed emotion and the increased relapse rate produced by this state of affairs is likely to tax the resources of most community services. The studies reported here do not show that relatives are less satisfied with the community services. The studies discussed here and by others also show reductions in admission rates. These two pieces of evidence might lead us to assume that the problem of expressed emotion itself is not one which needs much attention. These studies, however, occurred prior to the new financial limits and as Frank Holloway has pointed out this is likely to have major repercussions.

Families

As well as the problem of expressed emotion is the increased burden, both objective and subjective that is placed on the family. These stressors may lead to increased ill health in the main carers. Family burden has been addressed in many studies and it seems not to increase substantially. Even if the objective burden increases it does seem to produce a concomitant increase in subjective burden. Families are pleased to have a service which is responsive and where staff are aware of all their needs.

The community

There will be increases in community burden. General practitioners, in particular, have been voicing their worries over the increased burden they may be under following the many changes in health service legislation. People living in the users' community may also have to bear some responsibility as part of the caring community, for example neighbours and housing officers.

There may also be increases in violence and threats of violence in the community. In a study carried out in the 1960s and early 1970s the effect, over a 6-year period, of transferring patients to community oriented teams produced a statistically significant increase in the number of murders by people with mental illness compared with those with no such diagnosis (Grunberg *et al.*, 1977). Murder is not a very frequent occurrence and so it could take some time to amass a similar data set. It is likely that the community could be at more risk of violence or threats as the hospital based services are decreased. This is a very difficult area to assess in any evaluative study because it depends on reporting rates.

It is obvious that violence or threats are more likely to be reported to a community service which is more conspicuous than to a hospital based service. Trying to discover whether there has been an increase in public disturbance, especially in a control group of patients in a hospital based service, is likely to require far too many breaches of privacy for a study to be accepted by any ethical committee.

The media picture of patients in the community who are suffering from mental illness is one of being on the streets and causing problems and harassing law abiding, tax paying citizens. While this is not true, the problem is to overcome the visibility of disruptive clients. It will affect the acceptability of community care and the mobilisation of community resources.

We need a clear description of helpful and toxic characteristics to optimise our services. I would challenge the researchers from all the current studies to tell us not about their successes but about their failures.

Progress

A model community service with all its elements evaluated is a long way off but it is possible to access data from a number of different models over a number of years. One example of the build up of research and pragmatic data is the Hospital Hostels service. The first hostel was opened at the Maudsley and because of difficulties in finding an appropriate site it was situated at the edge of the Maudsley grounds. This was an initial criticism. Now it is clear from the other services which have moved from the hospital site that the hospital background provided a psychological back-up which was extremely helpful to staff. Other services have moved further from the hospital site, have reduced the numbers of staff or both. These services did not accept patients with severe disturbances or returned them to hospital. In one recently published study the patients got worse in terms of the increased levels of pro re nata (PRN) medication required, presumably to reduce behavioural disturbance (Allen *et al.*, 1993). The possibility of support although rarely called on was a psychological factor which may be crucial to running such a service.

Conclusions

All these criticisms or demands for more information do not help providers set up a service in their area. What is needed is a central register of key elements of community services and frequent reports of their failures and successes. No new drug would be allowed on the market without a system for the reporting of toxic side-effects. Community care needs its own system of yellow cards which may need to be anonymous to help the data collection.

I am particularly disappointed that the results of the randomised controlled trial have not yet dramatically changed the lives of people with mental health problems. We have tested a very narrow range of service models and most have been in urban or inner city surroundings in highly deprived areas. We should utilise the data we have so far by looking at more sensitive analyses.

Future studies should collect different data and, as usual, more of it. There is a need to identify the factors responsible for the success of particular service models. Most importantly, all possible toxic effects must be measured, including the effects on staff, patients, families and the community.

The lack of clear empirical data means that service providers must weigh up the pragmatic and clinical benefits against each other in the design of new services. Users may want to live in small houses with a few others but it may not be possible to provide specific specialist treatments in this sort of service organisation. We suspect that, in general, community treatments are no worse and no better than hospital based treatments. They may be cheaper, cost the same or be more expensive.

We have heard much in this volume about the successes of community care and very little about the failures. We need to be more candid about these failures because we may learn far more from them than we ever do from our successes.

References

Allen H, Baigent H, Kent A, Bolton J (1993). Rehabilitation and staffing levels in a 'new look' hospital hostel. *Psychological Medicine*, **23**: 203–11.

Boer H, Briscoe M (1992). Suicide prevention. *British Journal of Psychiatry*, **160**: 867 (letter).

Brown G (1989). Life events and their measurement. In Brown G, Harris T (eds) *Life Events and Illness*, pp. 3–46, Unwin and Hyman, London.

Cantor CH, Burnett PC, Quinn J, Nizette D, Brook C (1992). Suicide and community psychiatric care: preliminary report. *Acta Psychiatrica Scandinavica*, **85**: 229–33.

Dean C, Gadd EM (1990). Home treatment for acute psychiatric illness. *British Medical Journal*, **301**: 1021–3.

Fernando S, Storm V (1984). Suicide among psychiatric patients of a district general hospital. *Psychological Medicine*, **14**: 661–72.

Grunberg F, Klinger BI, Grumet B (1977). Homicide and deinstitutionalization of the mentally ill. Clinical and research reports. *Americal Journal of Psychiatry*, **134**: 685–7.

Koran LM, Sox HC, Marton KI *et al.* (1989). Medical evaluation of psychiatric patients. Results in a State Mental Health System. *Archives of General Psychiatry*, **46**: 733–40.

Kuipers E (1992). Expressed emotion research in Europe. *British Journal of Clinical Psychology*, **31**: 429–43.

Lazarus R, Folkman S (1984). *Stress, Appraisal and Coping*. Springer, New York.

Morgan H (1992). Suicide prevention: hazards on the fast lane to community care. *British Journal of Psychiatry*, **160**: 149–53.

Muijen M, Marks I, Connolly J, Audini B (1992). Home based care and standard hospital care for patients with severe mental illness: a randomised controlled trial. *British Medical Journal*, **304**: 749–54.

Santos AB, Deci PA, Lachance KR *et al.* (1993). Providing assertive community treatment for severely mentally ill patients in a rural area. *Hospital and Community Psychiatry*, **44**: 34–9.

Wing J, Cooper J, Sartorius N (1976). *Measurement and Classification of Psychiatric Symptoms: An Instruction Manual for the PSE and CATEGO Program*. Cambridge University Press, Cambridge.

Wykes T, Sturt E (1986). The measurement of social behaviour in psychiatric patients: an assessment of the reliability and validity of the SBS Schedule. *British Journal of Psychiatry*, **148**: 1–11.

Wykes T (1994). Predicting sympathetic and behavioural outcomes of community care. *British Journal of Psychiatry*, **165**: 486–92.

10

Community mental health services: towards an understanding of cost-effectiveness
MARTIN KNAPP

Policy context

The community care reforms introduced by the 1990 UK *National Health Service and Community Care Act* provide an important context for understanding the relevance and application of mental health service evaluations. They also generate or consolidate a number of demands for cost information and a better understanding of cost-effectiveness.

The 1990 reforms comprise a number of strategic changes (Social Services Inspectorate, 1992; Wistow *et al.*, 1994). They seek to alter the balance between institutional and community care, moving the emphasis away from long-term hospital provision in favour of care in the community and away from residential and nursing homes towards support in domiciliary settings. They stress the importance of decisions which are purchaser dominated rather than provider dominated and needs led rather than supply led. Care management and care programmes should be important elements in the new system, comprehensive assessment procedures should be adopted and users and carers given greater influence and choice. There will also be some shifting of responsibilities for decision-making and funding from the National Health Service (NHS) to local government. This will make it harder, for example, for health authorities to discharge hospital inpatients to residential or nursing homes without the agreement and funding of local authorities. Greater pluralism within the 'mixed economy of care' is encouraged.

These reforms are being introduced in pursuit of familiar, broad policy aims. For example, the community care White Paper, *Caring for People* (Cm 849, 1989), argued that these changes would improve user choice, service innovation and quality. It was also unequivocal in its emphasis on system cost-effectiveness. Cost awareness, if not cost

111

control, appears as an important national policy objective in the UK Government's recommendations for mental health services. Indeed, the cost dimension appears as early as the fourth paragraph in the *Mental Illness Handbook*, a supplement to *The Health of the Nation* White Paper (Cm. 1523, 1992). Later, the Handbook argued:

> In a situation where 'need is limitless and resources finite', organisation of the available resources is critical to ensure that allocations are used as cost-effectively as possible in order to provide the maximum possible health benefits
>
> *Department of Health, 1993, paragraph 1.9.*

The demand for cost information should come as no surprise. Planning in a top-down, provider led, single agency, public expenditure manner makes modest and uncomplicated demands on cost information systems and traditional line budgets are probably adequate in design and accessibility to satisfy most needs. But the *NHS and Community Care Act* requires health and social care decision-making to become bottom-up, needs led and multiple agency. It encourages innovations by introducing new financial and other incentives and its reforms make it more likely that system implications will be couched in terms of social and not merely public expenditures. In these new circumstances, policy-makers and planners need more and better cost information. Traditional line budgets were recognised as inadequate in the health service some years before the 1990 Act, so that the purchaser/provider split introduced by the reforms boosted changes which were already under way. In mental health care, with a number of agencies and professions involved, there is probably a need for new and broader data systems and also new attitudes.

Among the specific changes which precipitate a need for a clearer costs perspective are developments in macro-planning, case responsibilities and funding. The community care plans drawn up by local and health authorities will have to be affordable and their ramifications appreciated and accepted by all relevant agencies. The perverse incentives within the old system, which sometimes encouraged local and health authorities to minimise their own costs while simultaneously increasing someone else's costs (Audit Commission, 1986), are largely disappearing. Care management procedures will have their own cost information needs, particularly if budgetary responsibilities are devolved to fieldwork teams or individuals. The introduction of care programmes in the mental health field will bring new organisational costs, but may not have quite the same immediate information requirements, but a care programme which is drawn up without awareness of the ability of agencies to supply services and therefore awareness of the cost implications) is liable to run into difficulties (Schneider, 1995).

There are longer standing demands for costs data. Evaluating the implications of different and especially new policies and practices has sometimes meant looking at both outcomes and resources (e.g. Glass & Goldberg, 1977; Mangen *et al.*, 1983). Costs data are also needed for 'burden of illness' calculations (Davies & Drummond, 1993), the pricing of services for sale, either to clients and their relatives or to public authorities embarking on a policy of contracting out, and in the perennial performance reviews required for public probity, now often built around 'value for money audits' and 'efficiency scrutinies'.

In each case, whether new demands of the 1990s or longer established needs, the cost data requirements are rarely met. It is not the purpose of this chapter to offer detailed suggestions for the design of routine cost information systems to meet these demands. Rather, the aims are to suggest procedures for handling and interpreting costs data within evaluations, to illustrate their application and to tease out some of the policy and practice consequences. In these ways, our understanding of the cost-effectiveness of community mental health services might be enhanced.

Principles of cost evaluation

Economists have produced a number of 'good practice' guides to the examination of costs and the conduct of economic evaluations. One of the earliest and best within the health economics genre is Drummond's (1980) book on economic appraisal, subsequently extended with accounts of more recent evaluative tools (Drummond *et al.*, 1987). There is no equivalent in the mental health field, although Knapp & Beecham (1990) have recommended four basic principles for *costs* research which lie at the core of economic evaluation. These can guide studies of psychiatric policies, practices or programmes. They are used to structure the arguments and evidence presented in this chapter.

The first of these principles says that costs should generally be measured comprehensively, covering all relevant services and other financial implications. There are circumstances when exceptions can be made, as discussed below. There will be cost variations between service users, facilities and areas of the country. The second principle recommends examination of these variations for their policy and practice insights. Thirdly, like with like comparisons should be attempted: the influences of extraneous factors should be removed or qualifications made to ensure that comparable samples of users or facilities are studied. Finally, cost information should not stand alone: the fourth principle urges its integration with information on user and other outcomes. This ensures that we move from costs to cost-effectiveness. These four principles of cost evaluation are really no different in intent or adoption from the basic principles of a clinical evaluation. Although blind adherence would be inadvisable, the wider adoption of these principles should aid the policy and practice processes.

In order to move towards a clearer view of cost-effectiveness, and to discuss some of the issues confronting community mental health services, this chapter will draw on findings from three recent studies with which the Personal Social Services Research Unit (PSSRU) has been associated: the economic evaluations of the Daily Living Programme (DLP), an innovative community psychiatric nurse (CPN) service in Greenwich and the rundown of Friern and Claybury Hospitals in North London and psychiatric reprovision in the community. There are numerous other economic studies in the mental health area but property rights and familiarity make it easier to use these three evaluations to illustrate methodologies and arguments.

Comprehensive costs

Comprehensiveness in principle

Other things being equal, the greater and the more diverse a client's assessed needs, the broader the range of services likely to be utilised. The wider utilisation of comprehensive assessments in community settings and the purposive combination of services to meet needs are among the underlying principles of care management and care programming (North & Ritchie, 1993; Schneider, 1993). The influence of user choice and the extension of the mixed economy of health and social care will combine to broaden the range of services available in a locality and simultaneously to increase the variety of services used by individual people. An evaluation which addresses the resource dimension might therefore be called upon to cost a large number of services.

In many circumstances it would be necessary to cost every component of a care 'package'. There may be occasions when a particular evaluative trial is sufficiently narrow and when randomisation can guarantee the equivalence of some service utilisation so that inter-group comparisons can proceed without collecting costs data on everything. This is an approach suggested by Burns *et al.* (1993), for example. There might also be occasions when it is sufficient just to measure the most expensive elements in a set of services to gain a general indication of costs. This would not be sensible if the research seeks to illuminate *inter-individual differences* which, as argued below, is highly desirable within the context of the health and community care arrangements of the 1990s. A full costs picture will be needed in most instances.

There are obviously practical limits. It may be impossible within a research budget to identify every service used and the costing of forgone earnings and the burden of informal care on relatives and neighbours may itself be too costly. Evaluations of alternative forms of long-term care rarely will be able to run for as long as clients receive services before reaching definitive conclusions about relative costs. Nevertheless, costs measured over relatively short intervals could be used as the basis for extrapolation (see later). Psychiatric interventions for children and adolescents are particularly in need of a long-term perspective, given their potential lifetime effects (Knapp & Gilchrist, 1993).

The routinely quoted cost figures obtained from agency accounts are either total cost (actual expenditure on a service, usually during one financial year, perhaps with the addition of capital and charges for NHS facilities or a notional capital element for local authority facilities) or some measure of average cost (this total amount divided by a measure of workload, such as the number of patients seen). Economic theory would instead urge the use of marginal opportunity costs where 'marginal' refers to the addition to total cost attributable to the inclusion of one more patient and 'opportunity cost' refers to the opportunities forgone by not using a resource in its best alternative use. Opportunity costs give a truer measure of the private or social value of resources. The immediate cost of supporting one more person in a day care programme or accommodating one more resident in a hostel, the short-run marginal cost, may be small. If policy intentions are to substitute community services for all or most long-term hospital beds or to make other non-marginal adjustments to the balance of care, it makes no sense to use this short-term marginal measure as there is an obvious limit to the number of people who can be squeezed into existing services. Opportunity and marginal costs are described in more detail, for example, by Drummond (1980) and Knapp (1984, 1993).

Although the calculation and attachment of costs look complex, and although the principle of opportunity costing should never be abandoned, enthusiasm for it will have to be tempered when it comes to application. It happens that today's (short-run) average revenue cost (obtained from a complete set of agency accounts), plus appropriately measured capital and overhead elements, is probably close to the long-run marginal cost for many services used by people with mental health problems (Allen & Beecham, 1993). Moreover, there is now an excellent compendium of service costings, updated annually, which can greatly assist applied research (Netten & Smart, 1993). In all of the PSSRU studies described below, service utilisation data are collected using a variant of the Client Service Receipt Interview (CSRI; Beecham & Knapp, 1992).

Comprehensiveness in practice

The need for comprehensiveness is compelling when comparing hospital inpatient treatment with community based care because the former is almost all inclusive and the latter often comprises a multiplicity of services provided in different locations by different agencies. Savings from the rundown of hospitals are also expected to help fund the community services which replace them. Comprehensive cost comparisons between hospital and community services are therefore essential for planning and monitoring these financial transfers as well as for meaningful evaluation.

The process and outcome effects of the planned closure of Friern and Claybury psychiatric hospitals in North London are being studied by the Team for the Assessment of Psychiatric Services (TAPS; see Leff, 1993). The PSSRU is examining the costs. Most of the cost research to date has focused on the re-location of long stay inpatients (continuous hospital residence of 1 year or more) who, if aged over 65 years, do not have a current diagnosis of dementia. The patterns of service utilisation, cost and financing of psychiatric reprovision in the community 1 year after hospital discharge illustrate the importance of a comprehensive view (Hallam *et al.*, 1994; Knapp *et al.*, 1993).

Table 10.1 reports the most commonly-used services in the community. The table lists those services (out of a total of 40) which were used by more than 2% of the sample. Many agencies, departments and services are involved in supporting people with long-term mental health problems in the community. Although an average of 85% of total cost is accounted for by accommodation (including staff support provided within the place

Table 10.1 *Former Friern and Claybury Hospital inpatients: service utilisation in the community 1 year after discharge*

Selected services	Usage (%)	Contribution to cost	
		Users (%)	All (%)
Accommodation	100.0	84.9	84.9
General practitioner	80.4	0.4	0.4
Community psychiatry	60.4	0.6	0.4
Nursing	30.5	1.7	0.5
Hospital outpatient	25.2	1.9	0.4
Hospital inpatient	16.4	18.0	3.4
Hospital day patient	24.6	16.3	3.6
Social services department day care	22.0	7.9	1.8
Voluntary day care	19.4	7.1	1.5
Field social work	29.0	5.2	1.3
Education	5.6	6.9	0.5
Police	6.2	0.4	–

Sample size = 341 former inpatients (leavers cohorts 1 to 5).
Source: Knapp *et al.* (1993).

Table 10.2 *Former Friern and Claybury Hospital inpatients: funding contributions to community care*

Funding agency	Contribution to total cost (%)
District health authority	49.9
Family health service authorities	0.5
Local authority social services departments	9.9
Local authority housing departments	4.0
Other local authority departments	0.7
Voluntary sector	5.7
Social security/client	29.3
Total	100.0

Source: Knapp *et al.* (1993).

of residence), there are implications for other agencies and budgets. There is a high percentage use but low cost contribution for certain key services, such as general practice, community psychiatry and community nursing.[1] The funding consequences of these service use patterns can be seen in Table 10.2. At the time – prior to the introduction in April 1993 of the new funding route via local authority social services departments for financial support of long-term service users and the addition of community mental health services to the range of services purchased by general practitioners fundholders – half the total cost was borne by district health authorities and almost a third from social security payments to users or their places of residence.

With a multiplicity of services there are dangers if a comprehensive costs' perspective is not obtained. These dangers include the fragmentation of responsibilities, yawning gaps in service responsiveness to needs, underfunding of community care initiatives and cost shunting between agencies. Some of these problems are being addressed within the new arrangements for the management of finances and the support of users. Cost evaluations should not exacerbate these problems by deliberately omitting some services or budgets without good cause. This does not mean comprehensiveness at all cost; it simply means informed, often pragmatic, departures from the comprehensiveness principle.

Exploring variations

Variations in principle

Inter-client and inter-facility variations in cost are generally marked. They should not be ignored but should be explored for the policy and practice insights that they can often reveal. It is inappropriate to rely solely on averages for the purposes of evaluation and policy recommendations.

What causes the costs of community care to vary between individuals? Service or treatment responses reflect individual needs, albeit imperfectly. Because needs vary, so too will costs. Unless the organisation of community based care becomes so routine that it disregards individual needs, costs will partly reflect client differences. They will also reflect the preferences and perspectives of professionals and agencies, organisational scale and the characteristics of local communities and economies, for we know that some health and social care decision-making has been dominated by service availability. Another common source of cost variations is provider efficiency (Beecham *et al.*, 1991).

The number of potential influences on cost necessitates the use of multivariate statistical methods to explore variations. In some of the PSSRU research, we have used estimated statistical cost functions which have the advantages of strong roots in economic theory and accessible estimation routines. A disadvantage can be its need for a large data set, although the sample sizes usually employed in psychiatric evaluations will usually be sufficient. There is not the space to dwell on the conceptual r methodological details in this chapter (see Knapp, 1984, chapter 9; Knapp & Beecham, 1993*b*).

Variations in practice

his chapter offers three illustrations of the exploration of cost vari-
tions. The first examines the links between the characteristics of
ong-stay hospital inpatients and the subsequent costs of their care in
he community. Other potential cost raising factors occur *after* discharge
o a community setting and are considered later (the third of our cost
ariations explorations). Both of these examples build on the study of
he rundown of Friern and Claybury Hospitals. The second illustration
see later) comes from the evaluation of the DLP.

Data on the individual characteristics of hospital inpatients are col-
ected in interviews and assessments conducted by TAPS. Information
ncludes personal characteristics (sex, age, ethnic group, marital status,
npatient experience including length of stay, original diagnosis) and
letailed clinical, behavioural and social characteristics (O'Driscoll &
eff, 1993). The main instruments are: the Present State Examination
PSE, 9th edition; Wing *et al.*, 1974), the 1984 version of the Social
Behaviour Schedule (SBS; Sturt & Wykes, 1986), the Social Network
chedule (SNS; Dunn *et al.*, 1990; Leff *et al.*, 1990), the Physical Health
ndex (PHI; O'Driscoll & Leff, 1993), the Basic Everyday Living Skills
chedule (BELS; O'Driscoll & Leff, 1993) and the Patient Attitude
Questionnaire (PAQ; Thornicroft *et al.*, 1993). One aim of our study was
o develop a cost prediction equation which might assist service planners
o structure community support for people with long-term mental health
roblems leaving hospital.

The links between these hospital inpatient characteristics and subsequent costs in the community were examined in a series of ordinary
east squares regression equations, taking average weekly cost as the
lependent variable and introducing client characteristics as predictors.
The criteria for inclusion in the regression equations were statisti-
al significance, interpretability of estimated effects and parsimony.
Multivariate rather than bivariate analyses are needed to investigate
he simultaneous influences of different factors. The endstage equation
s summarised in Table 10.3 The overall statistical performance of the
egression analyses was quite good: estimates were robust (the removal
or addition of one variable did not throw the equation into chaos) and
he R-squared measure of goodness of fit (measuring the proportion of

Table 10.3 *Regression of community cost after 1 year on client characteristics in hospital prior to discharge*

Predictor variables	Coefficient	t-statistic	Significance
Constant	169.35	3.39	0.001
Male, divorced or separated[a]	143.86	2.65	0.009
Single[a]	75.47	2.73	0.007
Age in years, squared	–0.01	–1.69	0.093
Total previous time in mental hospital, in years, squared[b]	–0.09	–2.00	0.047
Percentage of life in hospital	543.33	2.82	0.005
Percentage of life in hospital, squared	–448.79	–1.73	0.084
Non-specific neurotic syndrome (PSE)	6.17	3.05	0.003
If male[a], delusions and hallucinations (PSE)	–4.22	–1.80	0.073
Negative symptoms (PSE)	23.07	2.56	0.011
Total Social Behaviour Schedule (SBS) score	28.50	3.00	0.003
Total SBS score, squared	–2.15	–2.64	0.009
If male[a], daily nursing care score, squared	77.50	2.34	0.020
Number of ex-patients named and seen (SNS)	–15.15	–1.71	0.089
Number of hospital staff named and seen	6.94	1.71	0.090
If male[a], total persons named and seen	–5.23	–3.31	0.001
R^2		0.35	
F-statistic		7.27	0.00

Sample size = 217.
[a] Dummy variable taking the value 1 if an individual has the named characteristic or diagnosis and the value 0 otherwise.
[b] Excludes current admission.
Source: Knapp *et al.* (1994a).

cost variation explained by the included variables) was a satisfactory 0.35. This indicates that one-third of the observed inter-client cost variation a year after discharge can be explained by reference to client characteristics before discharge from hospital. The equation is therefore useful for predictions of cost (it has the potential to perform better than non-statistical methods) and it contains some interesting associations, although a large part of the cost variation in the community is due to events which occur after discharge (see later).

It is possible to give only a brief interpretation of the effects contained within the estimated cost equation (for full details see Knapp *et al.*,

1994*a*). *Ceteris paribus*, the costs of community care are higher for people who:

never married (and also for the 6% of the sample who are divorced/separated men)
are older
are male
spent shorter periods in psychiatric hospitals (although the effect on cost is very small)
have spent greater proportions of their lives in hospital (although the effect is non-linear).

The influences of the clinical factors on cost are also interesting:

Three constructed PSE measures were significant: non-specific neurotic syndrome, negative symptoms and delusions and hallucinations. The first and second exerted positive effects, the third a negative effect, although only for males.

Higher scores on the SBS (greater staff reported ratings of abnormal behaviours) indicate higher needs and imply higher costs.

The greater the number of areas in which daily nursing care is required the higher are costs, although interestingly only for males.

The instrument used to gather data on social networks (the SNS) requires an interview with each patient. Schedules could not be completed for everyone. Higher SNS scores mean more social contacts. This usually means lower costs: more communicative and gregarious people are less costly. An exception is that hospital inpatients who saw more hospital staff later cost more in the community (although the effect is modest).

Diagnosis has no obvious effect on cost once the above factors have been taken into account. Diagnostic-related groups would therefore be of little predictive value for former long-stay hospital residents. It should be noted here that quality of life, health and welfare in the community for this sample of former long-stay inpatients were generally no worse than in hospital and in some respects significantly better (Anderson *et al.*, 1993). The links between outcomes and costs are addressed later.

The costs of community care 1 year after people left hospital can therefore be predicted, in part, by their needs and other personal characteristics in hospital. In a later section we briefly demonstrate how we might extrapolate from a prediction equation of this kind to a larger population.

Like with like comparisons

Comparisons in principle

The need to avoid spurious comparisons is as great in costs research as in any clinical evaluation and the methods employed to ensure like with like comparisons are similar. When circumstances allow, the randomised controlled trial should ensure comparability (although there might still be distortions and checks are advisable). Quasi-experimental designs with matched or statistical controls can also be employed. The route to statistical controls which we have used in our own research has followed the cost function approach mentioned earlier.

In adopting this third principle of applied costs research we are able to draw more confident conclusions about the resource implications of different ways of supporting people with mental health problems. Illustrations are given here of three different methodological approaches to like with like comparisons, picking up three different cost-effectiveness issues concerning community mental health services. The first examines alternative arrangements for a CPN service and employs a straightforward randomised controlled trial. The second describes the cost-effectiveness study of the DLP at the Maudsley, using the randomised controlled trial design as the basic framework for a more searching and informative investigation of the cost-raising effects of individual characteristics at the point of referral. The third returns to the Friern/Claybury study and uses a cost prediction equation to extrapolate to people and hospitals outside the sample of costed hospital leavers.

Comparisons in practice: alternative CPN arrangements

In 1989, the CPN service was reorganised in Greenwich, with individual staff acting as case managers and client advocates. This new arrangement was compared with the standard organisation of 'generic' CPN services in a controlled study by examining their activities and the associated costs and effects. Eighty-two people referred to the specialist psychiatric services by consultant psychiatrists or ward teams at the point of discharge from hospital (usually after short stays) or during community residence at the point at which CPN support was considered to be necessary met the study criteria (psychotic disorder, duration of illness of more than 2 years, more than two hospital admissions during the previous 2 years, aged 18–64 years). They were randomly allocated to either the traditional, generic CPN team or a new community support team (CST).

Tests revealed no significant differences between the two samples at entry to the study (Muijen *et al.*, 1994).

Each person was assessed four times: at entry to the study and after 6, 12 and 18 months. Data were gathered on clinical outcomes, social and behaviourial functioning, family burden and consumer satisfaction. At entry to the study, service use data were collected retrospectively for the previous 3 months. At subsequent interviews, service use data referred to the period since last interview. Data were also collected from case records on frequency and duration of CPN service receipt, including domiciliary and office visits and medication received. Muijen *et al.* (1994) report marked differences between the CST and generic CPN services in terms of the number and type of contacts but no differences in numbers of admissions, length of stay, social functioning, psychopathology or users' and relatives' satisfaction.

The economic evaluation found a difference in the weekly cost of all services and accommodation used between the two groups of clients in the study, with the generic (control) group costs 39% greater (£89 per week at 1989–90 prices) than the CST group, although the difference was only significant in the first 6 months of the evaluation period. In the longer term, the apparent cost differences were not significant: the 'care management' approach was no more or less cost-effective, although client satisfaction was slightly higher in the short term (Figure 10.1). The overall level of input from CPNs was significantly higher and more costly for the CST group and CPNs worked on a wider range of issues and areas (McCrone *et al.*, 1994). Unfortunately, the Greenwich CST evaluation was probably not long enough to test properly the ramifications of nurse based care management but it warrants attention because its aims are similar to some of the key proposals for the national development of community mental health services in the 1990s. The CPNs received no additional training but encouraging them to work with a wider range of responsibilities and services and giving them more autonomy produced some short-term economic advantages and no medium-term disadvantages. The CST model reduced reliance on specialist residential accommodation.

Comparisons in practice: the DLP

The DLP offered problem oriented, home based care for people with severe mental illness facing emergency admission to the Bethlem-Maudsley Hospital. As Marks describes in Chapter 3, the DLP was

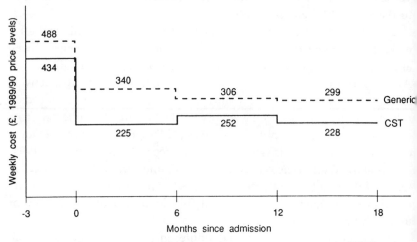

Figure 10.1 Greenwich CST initiative: average costs per week (McCrone *et al.*, 1994).

modelled on earlier experiments with intensive community support teams, particularly the community treatment programmes developed in Madison and Sydney. The multi-disciplinary DLP team acted as both direct provider and liaison with other services, with each person allocated a key worker.

Examination of the costs of the DLP and standard hospital based care was undertaken within a randomised controlled comparison (Knapp *et al.*, 1994*b*). The associations between costs in the final part of the evaluation period and the clinical, social and demographic characteristics of patients at admission were also examined. It can be seen from Figure 10.2 that the DLP was significantly less costly than standard treatment based initially on inpatient care in both the short and medium term (up to 20 months after admission). Reduced inpatient stays, however, were no longer a feature of DLP care in the longer term (30–45 months after trial admission) and, although the cost analyses await completion, there must be doubts as to the longer term cost implications.

In the short and medium terms, the cost advantage to the DLP, coupled with broadly encouraging outcome results over this period (Marks *et al.*, 1994), implies that the DLP was a cost-effective alternative to standard psychiatric care. Moreover, the DLP did not shift the burden of support and funding from the NHS to other agencies or to patients

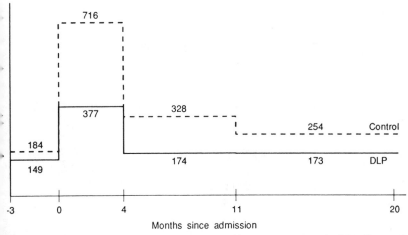

Figure 10.2 Daily Living Programme: average costs per week (Knapp *et al.* 1994*b*).

and families. Indeed, the costs of local authority social care services were slightly but significantly lower for the DLP than for the control group. Most of the cost savings associated with the DLP accrued to the NHS. Were the DLP to be a viable clinical procedure, these savings could create an incentive for further implementation.

The DLP evaluation allows the cost difference between experimental and control groups to be 'unpacked' by exploring the sources of within-sample cost variations. The first stage is to use a methodology identical to the approach used when predicting community costs for former Friern and Claybury Hospital inpatients. This involves examination of the links between characteristics at the point of referral and costs during the last of the evaluation periods (12–20 months after referral), looking at the DLP and control groups separately. This produced the final regression equations summarised in Table 10.4. The second stage is to conduct cross-predictions from these equations, which are described after first discussing the interpretation of the estimated equations.

The individual characteristics explored in the statistical analyses were constructed from assessments at entry to the study using the following instruments: the PSE (Wing *et al.*, 1974), the Global Assessment Scale (GF Endicott *et al.*, 1976), the Brief Psychiatric Rating Scale (BPRS; Overall & Gorham, 1962; Lukoff *et al.*, 1986), the Social Adjustment

Table 10.4 Cost prediction equations for the Daily Living Programme and control group samples[a]

Predictor variables	DLP sample			Control group		
	Coefficient	t	P	Coefficient	t	P
Constant	169.40	1.57	0.121	921.69	2.11	0.039
Female[b]	−62.51	−2.40	0.020			
Afro-Caribbean ethnic group[b]	99.41	3.06	0.003			
Lived with relatives at entry[b]	−86.64	−3.28	0.002			
Duration of previous inpatient admission (days)				6.68	1.97	0.053
Non-specific neurotic syndrome subscore[c] (PSE)	−14.84	−2.59	0.012			
Non-specific neurotic syndrome subscore[c], squared	0.45	2.38	0.021			
Delusions and hallucinations subscore[c] (PSE)	−12.43	−2.37	0.021	−0.40	−2.64	0.011
Delusions and hallucinations subscore[c], squared	0.42	1.75	0.085			
Specific neurotic syndrome subscore[c] (PSE), squared				0.76	1.86	0.067
BPRS score[c]				−36.18	−2.09	0.041
BPRS score[c], squared				0.37	2.27	0.027
SAS global score[c]	22.90	1.99	0.051			
SAS global score[c], squared	−0.60	−2.11	0.039	0.43	3.02	0.004
R^2	0.41			0.34		
F-statistic	4.47		0.000	5.26		0.000
n	68			68		

BPRS: Brief Psychiatric Rating Scale; PSE: Present State Examination; SAS: Social Adjustment Scale.
[a] Dependent variable is average weekly cost during the period 12–21 months after entry to the study (referral to the Maudsley), £, 1989/90 price levels.
[b] Dummy variable taking the value 1 if an individual has the named characteristic and the value 0 otherwise.
[c] Higher scores indicate more severe mental health problems.

Scale (SAS; Weissman *et al.*, 1971, 1974) and questions on clients' and relatives' satisfaction with services (Larsen *et al.*, 1979; Attkison & Zwick, 1985; Lemmens & Donker, 1990). Costs were measured using a version of the CSRI (Beecham & Knapp, 1992). Other characteristics which did not prove significant were age, Mental Health Act legal status and diagnosis. Both equations perform satisfactorily from a statistical viewpoint and both reveal interesting cost-need linkages.

For the control group, costs are higher in the medium term for people who scored more highly on the specific neurotic syndrome subscore of the PSE, the BPRS and the SAS global score. The only exception to the general finding of a positive link between needs at entry and costs between 12 and 20 months is the negative effect of the non-specific neurotic syndrome subscore of the PSE.

For the DLP group, the links between characteristics at entry and later costs are less straightforward. The non-specific neurotic syndrome and delusions and hallucinations subscores of the PSE and the SAS global score all exert curvilinear effects on average weekly cost. Greater needs at entry are *less likely* to be associated with higher costs for the DLP group than for the control group, which is probably an indication of the relative success of the DLP team in addressing mental health symptoms during this period (Marks *et al.*, 1994). Costs for the DLP group were also lower for females (a result also obtained in our NETRHA (Northeast Thames Regional Health Authority) study; Table 10.3), lower for the 64% of people who lived with relatives at entry (an indication, perhaps, of the DLP's ability to galvanise and support informal care) and higher for people in the Afro-Caribbean ethnic group (compare Thomas *et al.*, 1993). These analyses are not needed within a randomised controlled trial although they are themselves informative, for they provide an indication of the likely medium-term cost implications of people with different characteristics at entry (referral) and they hint at inter-individual differences in the future. Yet it is surprisingly rare to find studies that subject their data to this more searching interrogation.

These two multivariate analyses explore and standardise for differences *within* samples before drawing conclusions about cost raising characteristics. We can also use them to make cost comparisons *between* treatment options having standardised for individual differences. The research question is whether or to what extent the inter-group cost difference reflects differences in the characteristics of individuals or the consequences of different treatments. Cross-predictions can be made from the estimated equation fitted for one group to the actual characteristics of the other group. Using conventional notation, we can write the two cost prediction equations in Table 10.4 as:

$$C_{DLP} = \Sigma \beta_{DLP} X_{DLP} + U_{DLP}$$
$$C_{CTL} = \Sigma \beta_{CTL} X_{CTL} + U_{CTL}$$

In these equations, C denotes period or weekly cost, X the set of pre-sentence predictor variables, β the vector of estimated coefficients and U the residual. The subscripts DLP and CTL denote the two groups.

Using these equations we could predict or expect that, if the individuals who received standard inpatient treatment (control group service) had instead been supported by the DLP, their costs would be:

$$C_{CTL.DLP} = \Sigma \beta_{DLP} X_{CTL}$$

The predicted cost of the control group sample (denoted by the CTL subscript on the predicted cost C) had they received the DLP service (the DLP second subscript on C) is equal to the weighted sum of the control group characteristics X_{CTL}, with weights equal to the estimated coefficients from the DLP cost prediction equation, β_{DLP}. We are therefore taking the estimated DLP cost equation in Table 10.4 and predicting what costs would have been for members of the control group had they instead been DLP patients. A similar cross-prediction can be made from the corresponding control group cost equation into the DLP group.

The resultant predicted costs are given in Table 10.5. The costs on the leading diagonal (£178, £254) give the observed mean costs for the two groups[2]. The figures in the first row of the table indicate the costs of the two treatment options for the DLP group members. £178 is the observed mean weekly cost of DLP for the people who were actually allocated to the DLP service and £285 is the predicted cost for the same group if they had received standard inpatient treatment. If we compare vertically rather than horizontally, the figures in the first column give the predicted costs of receiving DLP for each of the two groups. Vertical comparisons reflect differences in group characteristics. The difference between the mean costs of each pair of groups/treatments can be decomposed into a functional component (the effect of the treatment) and a characteristics component (the effect of the individual). For example, the simple difference between the costs of standard inpatient treatment and DLP, is:

$$\bar{C}_{DLP} - \bar{C}_{CTL} = \Sigma \beta_{DLP} X_{DLP} - \Sigma \beta_{CTL} X_{CTL}$$

Table 10.5 *Predicted weekly costs, DLP evaluation*

Sample	Predicted costs for treatment types		
	DLP	Standard	Significance
DLP			
Mean	£178	£285	0.001
SD	£123	£236	
Standard (control)			
Mean	£196	£254	0.096
SD	£93	£259	
Significance	0.175	0.297	

DLP: Daily Living Programme; SD: standard deviation.

Without altering the total on the right hand side, we can add and subtract the predicted mean for the standard inpatient treatment group had they received DLP treatment:

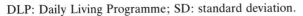

$$\bar{C}_{DLP} - \bar{C}_{CTL} = (\Sigma \beta_{DLP}X_{DLP} - \Sigma \beta_{DLP}X_{CTL}) + (\Sigma \beta_{DLP}X_{CTL} - \Sigma \beta_{CTL}X_{CTL}$$

The first parenthesis contains a measure of the cost difference attributable to individual differences (those found in the DLP function). The second parenthesis contains a measure of the 'real difference' in costs on a like with like basis. The results of this decomposition yield the following:

$$-76 = (178-254) = (178-196) + (196-254) = (-18) + (-58)$$

Thus DLP's simple cost advantage of £76 over standard inpatient treatment decomposes into a difference of only £18 per week due to differences in the characteristics of the samples ($P=0.175$) and a real difference in treatment cost of £58 ($P=0.096$). If we use the standard inpatient treatment function as the basis for decomposition, we find an inter-sample difference of £31 ($P=0.297$) due to individual characteristics and a true (like with like) cost advantage to DLP of £107 ($P=0.001$). Costs are expressed at 1989–90 price levels.

These results therefore have three important implications. Firstly, there are no significant cost raising differences between the DLP and control group samples. Secondly, there are significant differences between

DLP and standard inpatient treatment costs. Removing the small individual effect, we find the DLP treatment to be either £58 or £107 per week cheaper in the medium term (12–20 months after entry), on average some 32% lower than standard treatment based initially on inpatient care. Thirdly, closer examination of the estimated equations shows that the costs of the DLP are lower than standard care (in the medium term) for all admissible values of the indicators for the SAS, BPRS, delusions and hallucinations and specific neurotic syndrome (PSE) and for virtually all admissible values of the non-specific neurotic syndrome (PSE) indicator. In other words, the DLP cost advantage in the medium term applies to virtually all levels and types of need covered by the study.

Comparisons in practice: hospital closure extrapolations

The third like with like comparison uses the examination of links between characteristics of Friern and Claybury inpatients and their subsequent community care costs to extrapolate to later leavers, to other hospitals and even nationally.

Almost all community resettlement schemes have begun by first moving rather less dependent people from hospital. This is sensible as the development of good community services takes time and involves personal, professional and political risks. The risks will be fewer for those patients whose needs are more easily met. In the Friern and Claybury case, early movers to the community 'were significantly younger, had spent less time in full-time psychiatric care, were less likely to have a diagnosis of schizophrenia, had larger social networks and were more likely to want to leave hospital' (Jones, 1993, p.36). They also had fewer behavioural problems and were less likely to suffer from delusions and hallucinations. The differences between early movers and stayers as a result of this selective resettlement process, combined with what we know about the community cost consequences of different inpatient characteristics (as reported above), however, have caused the average cost for successive cohorts of leavers to rise (Table 10.6).

The research problem is the difficulty of generalising from the first people rehabilitated from hospital to later leavers. Certainly, comparisons of today's inpatient and community care average costs will probably not be comparing like with like. The policy problems caused by this 'cream skimming' include the danger of underfunding the expansion of community care and the observation that the costs of both hospital and community care appear to be rising.[3]

Table 10.6 *Reprovision for long-stay psychiatric hospital inpatients: costs after 1 year in the community by annual cohort of leavers*

			Cost per week (£)[a]		
Cohort	Year of leaving	Year of costing	Mean	SD	Sample size
1	1985/86	1986/87	246	101	43
2	1986/87	1987/88	366	171	110
3	1987/88	1988/89	421	175	115
4	1988/89	1989/90	357	202	74
5	1989/90	1990/91	465	193	148
6	1990/91	1991/92	552	159	55
1–6	1985–91	1986–92	413	192	545

[a] At 1989–90 price levels.
Source: Hallam *et al.* (1994).

These problems of valid comparisons can be illustrated with the help of Figure 10.3. The two lines in the figure represent the average costs of hospital provision and community care as an increasing function of 'dependency' (a general term used to denote the symptoms of mental ill health, behavioural problems, nursing care needs, social networks, etc; alternatively, the generic term 'need' could be used). The assumption of a positive cost-dependency relationship is justified by reference to the estimated function in Table 10.3 (for dependency relationship is justified by reference to the estimated function in Table 10.3 (for community care) and by less detailed evidence for hospitals (Knapp & Beecham, 1990). It has also been assumed that the cost of hospital care is lower than the cost of community care for some people, usually those who are very dependent, an assumption supported by the data in this NETRHA study and in other research (e.g. Häfner & an der Heiden, 1989). Finally it is assumed that the 'average degree of dependency (or ill health)' of people *currently* accommodated in hospital is greater than the average in the community, an assumption that accords with anecdotal evidence but cannot easily be verified statistically.

Today's observed mean costs of hospital and community care thus reflect differences in both the locus of care or treatment and the people supported. If someone of average dependency within the hospital population moves to the community, the expected community cost will not be the present average community cost (denoted *C* in Figure 10.3) but the higher amount *M*. The total savings realised by moving people from hospital to community care, therefore, will be exaggerated by the simple

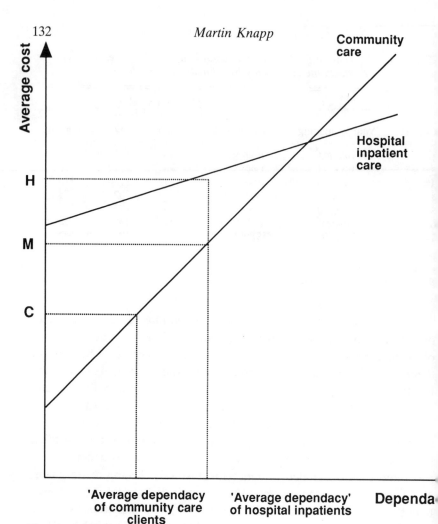

Figure 10.3 Long-stay psychiatric inpatient care and community re-provision costs and dependency.

(mean) average cost figures prepared for clients *currently* in care (even if these costs were comprehensively measured). The average saving is not $H-C$ but $H-M$. This illustrates the danger of the underfunding of community care initiatives.

When someone of dependency which is less than the hospital average but *greater* than the community average moves from hospital to community, as often happens (Jones, 1993), there will be an increase in the (mean) average cost of both services. The mean hospital cost will rise because one of the less dependent inpatients has left and the mean community cost will rise because someone more dependent than the average has arrived. Despite this real cost inflation in both settings, total expenditure will fall. This helps to explain the real cost inflation experienced by both hospital and community services in the past few years.[3] As an increasingly large proportion of the hospital population moves into community provision, the differences in average dependency and cost will narrow as the populations become more alike.

This simple analysis, which is built on assumptions which appear to be valid under today's circumstances, reveals problems of research interpretation and care planning. In the NETRHA case, we endeavoured to use the estimated function linking costs in the community 1 year after discharge to user characteristics *prior* to discharge to give us a single linking function that cuts through the problem of the two lines in Figure 10.3.[4] The equation in Table 10.3 is an example. An earlier version was used to extrapolate to the full long-stay populations of Friern and Claybury to predict the full costs of psychiatric re-provision in the community for long-stay inpatients without dementia (Knapp *et al.*, 1990).[5]

We concluded from those early extrapolations that, in the long term, the money released by hospital closures should be sufficient to cover the costs of community care of all long-stay residents without dementia, although the financial burden will not be equally distributed between agencies. In particular, there must be concern as to the ability of local authorities to provide sufficient community care services given the growing demands upon them and the often parlous fiscal state of local government. Although we have not repeated in full these earlier projections of community care costs for the long-stay psychiatric hospital population, we have yet to find evidence to change our broad conclusion.[6]

Merging costs and outcomes

Costs and outcomes in principle

Central to the development of community mental health services must be a better understanding of the effects of service interventions on client welfare (the outcome question) and the associated resource implications (the cost question). The links between outcomes and costs must also be appreciated. To state the glaringly obvious, outcomes constitute one side of the cost-effectiveness relationship. However, it is rare for cost figures to be quoted alongside information on client outcomes or effectiveness, partly because the latter are difficult to define and measure and partly because accountants, treasurers and other custodians of financial information have rarely had the incentive, encouragement or opportunity to examine the wider picture. In the broad scheme of things, there is no more justification for this than for conducting an outcome study without any idea of the resource implications of the options being studied.

Economic evaluations take three main forms when examining cost-outcome links: cost-effectiveness analysis (CEA), cost-benefit analysis (CBA) and cost-utility analysis (CUA) (Drummond, 1980; Knapp, 1984, chapters 7, 8; Maynard, 1993). They share six common stages: definition of the alternatives to be examined; listing of costs and outcomes; quantification and valuation of costs and outcomes; comparison of costs and outcomes; qualification or revision of the comparison in the light of risk, uncertainty and sensitivity (to assumptions); and examination of the distributional implications. The last of these is necessary if, as is often the case, the primary purpose of an evaluation is the examination of efficiency.[7]

At the third stage the analyses take different approaches: a CUA seeks to reduce outcomes to a single dimension by employing appropriate weights gleaned from empirical work or elsewhere, a CBA uses monetary weights to aggregate the outcomes and a CEA sticks with single or multiple outcomes measured using corresponding scales and indicators. With a CEA, the decision rule would be to compare the costs of obtaining levels of outcome and to conclude that the option with lowest cost per given level of outcome is the more efficient. This is obviously not easy to apply in practice, particularly with multi-dimensional outcome measures that do not move in concert. If some outcome dimensions register improvements and others deteriorate, or if the cost and outcome comparisons point to different preferred solutions, the decision rule may be difficult to implement.

CEA is therefore of most value when 'choosing between mutually exclusive ways of achieving a particular, very clearly defined benefit' (Sugden & Williams, 1978, p.191). It cannot be used to say whether the benefits of a project or procedure actually outweigh the costs. On the other hand, a CEA can ensure that a full range of costs is estimated and that measures are sought for all relevant dimensions of outcome and it does so without introducing all of the difficulties and additional value judgements associated with the attachment of monetary values to outcomes. It is not the responsibility of the analyst/researcher to decide on a particular policy or treatment; trading off costs against outcomes must be the responsibility of the policy-maker. It is the task of the analyst to lay out the various consequences with sufficient detail and clarity for informed decisions to be made.

CUA is a cost-effectiveness analysis conducted with outcomes measured by 'utility', the best-known example in health care evaluations being the use of QALYs (quality-adjusted life years). The QALY is the weighted aggregate of scores measuring pain and disability. With a CUA it is possible (although not always sensible) to calculate and compare the cost per unit of utility for different clinical procedures or even different social problems (e.g. comparing kidney transplants with treatment of cystic fibrosis with cetfazidime; Gudex, 1990). Although the QALY provides decision-makers with a set of precise looking statistics, and in so doing has contributed enormously by concentrating clinicians' and managers' minds on the thorny issues of resource allocation and priorities, there are some difficulties and dangers. As well as the obvious technical challenges of obtaining the weights to trade one dimension off against another, there is also the danger of loss of information when many outcome dimensions are squeezed into a uni-dimensional straitjacket (Donaldson *et al.*, 1988; Loomes & McKenzie, 1989; Carr-Hill & Morris, 1991). The QALY has rarely been examined in mental health contexts (Wilkinson *et al.*, 1990; discussed in Knapp & Kavanagh, 1992).

These three modes of economic evaluation combining information on costs and outcomes can be embellished, and often considerably enhanced, with a supplementary cost function. The cost function was introduced earlier. In its fully specified form it is the estimated relationship between the cost of providing a service or programme of support, user and other outcomes, input prices and other factors with an hypothesised influence on cost. The precise form of a cost function is determined by the interaction of *a priori* theoretical considerations and statistical findings. It can be interpreted as a multivariate version of the CEA, CBA, or CUA.

There are two circumstances when the cost function is particularly useful. When randomisation is not possible, it provides a means of statistical matching which was effectively what we were doing in the extrapolation of community care costs to hospital inpatients (see earlier). Secondly, when it is believed that the differences between individuals and/or the services they receive are sufficiently great to warrant examination of the impact of different combinations of individual characteristics and service packages on cost and/or outcome, the cost function provides the means to unpack the variations. This was the rationalisation for its use in the

135

 ̧multivariate analyses of the DLP data. This is what we
 ̦havioural cost function, estimated with the individual client
 ̹vice as the unit of analysis, whose interpretation will need
 ̧s much from psychology and sociology as from economics.

Costs and outcomes in practice

Thᴇ ᵥ ᴎplest integration of costs and outcomes has already been alluded
to when describing the three studies which illustrate the methods of
cost evaluation. For example, the outcome evaluation of the Greenwich
initiative, with CPNs performing roles which approach those usually
associated with care or care management, found no differences between
control and experimental groups in relation to the number or duration of
inpatient admissions, scores on the main instruments measuring clinical
characteristics and social functioning (SAS, GAS, BPRS, PSE), or users'
and relatives' satisfaction (Muijen *et al.*, 1994). The cost evaluation found
the generic (control) CPN arrangement to be 39% more expensive
than the new CST arrangement group, although significantly different
only in the first 6 months (McCrone *et al.*, 1994). The CST model is
therefore a short-term cost-effective alternative to standard, generic
CPN services, although the cost-effectiveness advantage disappears in
the medium term. There is no difficulty in combining the different
outcomes for they all register the same result: no difference between
the two groups.

Similar simple combinations of the results from the outcome and cost
evaluations for the Maudsley DLP would lead us to conclude that the
DLP was a cost-effective alternative to standard hospital based care
for people with serious mental health problems in the first 21 months
after admission. Symptoms and social adjustment were improved, the
expressed satisfaction of clients and relatives was significantly higher and
costs were lower (Knapp *et al.*, 1994*b*; Marks *et al.*, 1994).

There should be no doubts about the validity of these cost-effectiveness
methodologies, and the results they produce may be of policy significance, but they do not fully exploit the opportunities offered by the data.
As argued above, even with a randomised controlled design, there could
be merit in examining inter-individual differences for the revelations they
can offer for policy and practice. Armed with good outcome data, a
cost function analysis can separate the links between resource utilisation
(as summarised by cost) and the outcomes which result, while holding
constant the influences of relevant covariates.

An illustration of this methodology is offered by the NETRHA study of community reprovision for long-stay psychiatric hospital inpatients.[8] Employing data for members of just the first three annual cohorts of leavers, we examined the factors which together best explained the observed variation in weekly cost of community care 1 year after discharge from hospital (Beecham *et al.*, 1991). Unlike the earlier examination of the predictive power of inpatient characteristics (see earlier), the full cost function allows the introduction of measures of outcomes and community needs. The latter are measured by the scores on the instruments used to assess people 1 year after leaving hospital and the former by the differences between these scores and the corresponding scores at the time of the assessment in hospital. Other variables examined in the cost function include certain characteristics of the community care environments.

The cost function was estimated by ordinary least squares multiple regression, its final representation being selected on the usual criteria of statistical significance, interpretability and parsimony (Table 10.7). In fact, two estimated cost functions are reported, one of them excluding the dummy variables for sector of accommodation (private, voluntary, local authority, health authority). They explain 57% and 64% of the observed community cost variation, a considerable improvement on the equation predicting costs only from hospital characteristics (Table 10.3).[9] It is not necessary to discuss every one of the factors shown to have a significant effect on costs but some key findings should be emphasised.

The first is that there is an encouragingly strong link between costs and outcomes. Higher community care costs (higher levels of spending) were associated with greater improvements in the health and welfare of former hospital inpatients. In particular, improvements in negative symptoms, delusions and hallucinations, social networks (broadening) and the general need for care (from an index of physical health) are all associated with higher costs. These positive cost-outcome links are consistent with earlier findings (Knapp *et al.*, 1992b).

A second key finding is that costs are sensitive to client characteristics and needs (as assessed in the community). Costs are higher for people with blunting of affect, incontinence, mobility problems and community living skills. Community care services are being targeted with at least some success. Another finding to note from this estimated cost function is that the private and voluntary sectors appear to be able to provide community care services for former long-stay inpatients more cost-effectively than local authorities, who in turn are more cost-effective than health

Table 10.7 *Estimated cost functions (NETRHA psychiatric reprovision study)*

	Equation A		Equation B	
	Coefficient	Significance[c]	Coefficient	Significance
Constant term	37.0		131.2	***
Client never married[a]	54.3	***	53.4	***
Length of stay in hospital (months)	0.211	***	0.118	**
Community skills (BELS)	19.0	**		
Community skills, squared	-1.36	***	-0.385	***
Activity and social relationships (BELS)	8.59	***	7.82	***
Blunting of affect (PSE)	59.1	***	53.4	***
Incontinent (PHI)[a]	72.7	***	71.8	***
Impaired mobility (PHI)[a]	83.7	**	74.1	**
Social network: patients (SNS) squared	1.37	***	1.16	***
Expressed desire to move (PAQ)	54.6	**	44.8	**
Absolute difference in negative symptoms (PSE)	-22.3	***	-14.3	**
Relative difference in general anxiety squared (PSE)	14.0	***	12.3	***
Relative difference in delusions, hallucinations (PSE)	-0.123	***	-0.08	*
Reduced need for care (PHI)[a]	150		117	**
Absolute difference in non-professional network (SBS)	3.55	**	3.34	***

Table 10.7 (*cont.*)

	Equation A		Equation B	
	Coefficient	Significance[c]	Coefficient	Significance
Relative difference in relatives network (SNS)	−0.360	***	−0.278	**
Relative difference in patient network (SNS)	−0.207	**		
Improved helpfulness of medication (PAQ)	72.7	**	70.2	**
Health authority accommodation	NI		58.8	***
Voluntary or private sector accommodation	NI		−44.8	**
R^2	0.568	***	0.642	***
Adjusted R^2	0.499		0.585	

Sample size = 132.

NI: indicates variable not included in the set of possible regressors.

[a] Dummy variable taking the value 1 if the condition is satisfied, 0 otherwise.

[b] The instruments are listed and referenced in the text.

[c] Significance levels from t-tests on individual coefficients are F-test on goodness of fit (R^2): *** $P \leq 0.01$, ** $0.01 < P \leq 0.05$, * $0.05 < P \leq 0.10$.

authorities. A fuller discussion of the details of these results is given in Beecham *et al.* (1991).

Towards an understanding of cost-effectiveness

A number of questions about the viability, affordability and cost and outcome implications of a policy of community mental health care remain unanswered. Nevertheless, as argued in this chapter, relevant and illuminating research methodologies are in place, even if some of them (particularly the multivariate analysis of inter-individual differences) have been employed less often than one would like. It should be clear that cost research need not be the horrendous, ideologically compromising or scientifically complex task that some people appear to fear. On the other hand, there are examples of bad costs research to demonstrate that it is not as straightforward as some (other) people may have thought. It is encouraging that there is not a relatively large amount of health economics research focused on mental health services and programmes.

No attempt has been made in this chapter to summarise all available UK evidence,[10] although economists' answers to some of the important policy and practice questions are now being offered.

For the long-stay populations of England's psychiatric hospitals,[11] the study of the rundown of Friern and Claybury Hospitals, based on cost-prediction equations and extrapolations for inpatients without dementia, suggests that the savings from closing hospital provision should be adequate to fund community care services of at least equivalent quality. The funds for community care services must be transferred *before* hospitals can release them in order to finance capital investment, recruit staff and set support networks in place. The funds must also be allocated appropriately, which at the moment means getting more resources to local authority mental health services. There is also an obvious need for better coordination and joint action between the various parts of the statutory and non-statutory sectors, in both case planning and area planning.

For people with acute mental health problems, there is evidence that treatment or care in the community can be less costly than hospital inpatient care. The evaluations completed to date have found small but sometimes significant improvements in client circumstances and satisfaction for the experimental, largely community based services when compared with the standard, largely hospital based services. There is not yet evidence that this cost-effectiveness advantage is preserved over the longer term. Completed evaluations also point to interesting cost and outcome differences between alternative arrangements of community care. Even if the available evidence was exploited fully, the cumulative UK evidence on cost-effectiveness still does not amount to a great deal and the conclusion which should dominate all others is that one must be wary of generalisations which stray too far beyond the boundaries of completed research.

Acknowledgements

This chapter is based on a paper presented at the Department of Health *Review of Community Psychiatric Services*, London, March 1993, in turn based on two chapters of a forthcoming edited book (Knapp, 1995). Some of the material reported in this chapter is based on research undertaken at the PSSRU and in collaboration with researchers elsewhere, as citations indicate, and I am grateful to my colleagues Jeni Beecham, Andrew Fenyo, Angela Hallam and Vivien Koutsogeorgopoulou for their support, advice and permission to use jointly completed work. (This paper is lodged as PSSRU Discussion Paper 925/2.)

Notes

1 Five services account for 94% of total cost and ten services for 98%. This is a helpful finding, for it suggests that concentration on just a few services would produce cost estimates for the group which are close to the true (full) service and living costs of community care. Such a 'reduced list' method can therefore cut the costs of doing costs research, although it would not be appropriate for analyses at the individual level (Knapp & Beecham, 1993a). *Ceteris paribus*, a small number of services will account for a high proportion of total cost when staffed accommodation is heavily used, when evaluating programmes for people with chronic mental health problems and when community care 'packages' follow a few set patterns.

2 The figures reported in the table are calculated only for those patients for whom we have the information necessary to estimate the cost prediction equations. These figures will therefore differ slightly from those for the full samples reported above, which were calculated regardless of the availability of non-cost data.

3 Irrespective of this 'creaming' process, hospital cost inflation is inevitable during a process of rundown towards eventual closure as (quasi-fixed) overhead costs have to be spread across smaller numbers of inpatients.

4 We could not fit a function linking characteristics of inpatients to hospital costs because we did not have individualised hospital cost data. These data are difficult to collect at a disaggregated level and difficult to allocate to individual people when hospitals are moving towards closure because staff and patients tend to get moved between wards.

5 National extrapolations to the rest of England were also hazarded (Knapp *et al.*, 1992*a*).

6 With Friern Hospital now closed and our NETRHA-funded research continuing, we will be able to calculate actual rather than extrapolated costs. We are also looking at the costs of reprovision for acute and psychogeriatric inpatients.

7 There is always the danger that the distributional findings, and equity more generally, might get subsumed under and dominated by efficiency and there is also the danger that a CEA or other analysis becomes a vehicle for the analyst's or sponsor's own prejudices. Thus, while it would be wrong for the analyst not to make clear the implications of alternatives for individuals in different socio-economic groups, in different areas of the country or with different needs, it would be equally wrong to give the treatment of the distributional consequences any scientific, value-free veneer.

8 We have yet to complete the full set of cost-outcome analyses for the DLP evaluation. The Greenwich samples may be too small for full cost function exploration.

9 The prediction equation from hospital characteristics which corresponds to the cost function in Table 7, that is, the equation estimated for only the first three annual cohorts of leavers – explained 39 per cent of the observed variation in community care costs.

10 O'Donnell (1991) provides the most recent summary and review of UK evidence.

11 We are currently also looking at community care as an alternative to long-stay psychiatric hospital residence in Northern Ireland and, shortly, in Scotland.

References

Allen C, Beecham J (1993). Costing services: ideals and reality. In: Netten A, Beecham J (eds) *Costing Community Care: Theory and Practice*, pp. 25–42, Ashgate, Aldershot.

Anderson J, Dayson D, Willis W *et al* (1993). Clinical and social outcomes of long-stay psychiatric patients after one year in the community. *British Journal of Psychiatry* **162** (Suppl. 19): 45–56.

Attkison CC, Zwick R (1985). The Client Satisfaction Questionnaire: psychometric properties and correlation with service utilization and psychotherapy outcome. *Evaluation and Program Planning*, **5**: 233–7.

Audit Commission (1986). *Making a Reality of Community Care*. HMSO, London.

Beecham J, Knapp MRJ (1992). Costing psychiatric interventions. In: Thornicroft G, Brewin C, Wing J (eds.) *Measuring Mental Health Needs*, Oxford University Press, Oxford.

Beecham J, Knapp MRJ, Fenyo A (1991). Costs, needs and outcomes. *Schizophrenia Bulletin*, **17**: 427–39. Reprinted in: Netten A, Beecham J, (eds) *Costing Community Care: Theory and Practice*, pp. 162–76, Ashgate, Aldershot.

Burns T, Raftery J, Beadsmoore A, McGuigan S, Dickson M (1993). A controlled trial of home based acute psychiatric services. II. Treatment patterns and costs. *British Journal of Psychiatry*, **163**: 55–61.

Carr-Hill R, Morris J (1991). Current practice in obtaining the 'Q' in QALY's: a cautionary note. *British Medical Journal*, **303**: 699–701.
Cm 849 (1989). *Caring for People*. HMSO, London.
Cm 1523 (1992) *Health of the Nation*. HMSO, London.
Davies LM, Drummond MF (1993). Assessment of costs and benefits of drug therapy for treatment-resistant schizophrenia in the United Kingdom. *British Journal of Psychiatry*, **162**: 38–42.
Department of Health (1993). *Mental Illness Handbook (of the Health of the Nation)*. HMSO, London.
Donaldson C, Atkinson A, Bond J, Wright KG (1988). Should QALYs be programme specific? *Journal of Health Economics*, **7**: 239–57.
Drummond MF (1980). *Principles of Economic Appraisal in Health Care*. Oxford Medical Publications, Oxford.
Drummond M, Stoddart GL, Torrance GW (1987). *Methods for the Economic Evaluation of Health Care Programmes*. Oxford Medical Publications, Oxford.
Dunn M, O'Driscoll C, Dayson D et al. (1990). An observational study of the social life of long-stay patients. *British Journal of Psychiatry*, **157**: 842–8.
Endicott J, Spitzer RL, Fleiss JL, Cohen J (1976). The Global Assessment Scale. A procedure for measuring overall severity of psychiatric disturbance. *Archives of General Psychiatry*, **33**: 766–71.
Glass NJ, Goldberg D (1977). Cost-benefit analysis and the evaluation of psychiatric services. *Psychological Medicine*, **7**: 701–7.
Gudex C (1990). The QALY: how it can be used. In: Baldwin S, Godfrey C, Propper C (eds) *Quality of Life: Perspectives and Policies*, Routledge, London.
Häfner H, Heiden W an der (1989). Effectiveness and cost of community care for schizophrenic patients. *Hospital and Community Psychiatry*, **40**: 59–63.
Hallam A, Beecham J, Knapp MRJ, Fenyo A (1994). The costs of accommodation and care: community provision for former long-stay psychiatric hospital patients. *European Archives of Psychiatry and Clinical Neuroscience*, **243**: 301–10.
Jones D (1993). The selection of patients for re-provision. *British Journal of Psychiatry*, **162**: (Suppl. 19): 36–9.
Knapp MRJ (1984). *The Economics of Social Care*. Macmillan, London.
Knapp MRJ (1993). Background theory. In: Netten A, Beecham J (eds) *Costing Community Care: Theory and Practice*, pp. 9–24, Ashgate, Aldershot.
Knapp MRJ (ed.) (1995). *The Economic Evaluation of Mental Health Services*. Ashgate, Aldershot (in press).
Knapp MRJ, Beecham J (1990). Costing mental health services. *Psychological Medicine*, **20**: 893–908.
Knapp MRJ, Beecham J (1993a). *Reduced-list costings: examination of an informed short cut in mental health research*. Discussion Paper 939, Personal Social Services Research Unit, University of Kent at Canterbury.
Knapp MRJ, Beecham J (1993b). Health economics and psychiatry: the pursuit of efficiency. In: Bhugra D, Leff J (eds) *Principles of Social Psychiatry* pp. 549–61. Blackwell Scientific Publications, Oxford.
Knapp MRJ, Beecham J, Anderson J et al. (1990). Predicting the community

costs of closing psychiatric hospitals. *British Journal of Psychiatry*, **157**: 661–70.

Knapp MRJ, Beecham J, Fenyo A, Hallam A (1994*a*). Predicting costs from needs and diagnoses: community mental health care for former hospital inpatients. *British Journal of Psychiatry* (in press).

Knapp MRJ, Beecham J, Gordon K (1992*a*). Predicting the community costs of closing psychiatric hospitals: national extrapolations. *Journal of Mental Health*, **1**: 315–25.

Knapp MRJ, Beecham J, Hallam A, Fenyo A (1993). The costs of community care for former long-stay psychiatric hospital residents. *Health and Social Care*, **1**: 193–201.

Knapp MRJ, Beecham J, Koutsogeorgopoulou V *et al.* (1994*b*). Service use and costs of home based versus hospital based care for people with serious mental illness. *British Journal of Psychiatry*, **165**: 195–203.

Knapp MRJ, Cambridge P, Thomason C, Beecham J, Allen C, Darton R (1992*b*). *Care in the Community: Challenge and Demonstration*. Ashgate, Aldershot.

Knapp MRJ, Gilchrist S (1993). *Long-term costs of anti-social behaviours: issues for child psychiatry*. Discussion Paper 940, Personal Social Services Research Unit, University of Kent at Canterbury.

Knapp MRJ, Kavanagh S (1992). Health economics relevant to developments in community psychiatry. *Current Opinion of Psychiatry*, **5**: 314–19.

Larsen DH, Attkison CC, Hargreaves WA, Nguyen TD (1979). Assessment of client/patient satisfaction: development of a general scale. *Evaluation and Program Planning*, **2**: 197–207.

Leff J, (ed.) (1993). The TAPS Project: evaluating community placement of long-stay psychiatric patients. *British Journal of Psychiatry*, **162**, (Suppl.).

Leff J, O'Driscoll C, Dayson D *et al.* (1990). The TAPS Project. 5. The structure of social-network data obtained from long-stay patients. *British Journal of Psychiatry*, **157**: 848–52.

Lemmens F, Donker, M (1990). Kwaliteitsbeoordeling door clienten. Utrecht, *Nederlands Centrum Geestelijke Volksgezondheid*.

Loomes G, McKenzie L (1989). The use of QALY's in health care decision making. *Social Science and Medicine*, **28**: 299–308.

Lukoff D, Liberman RP, Neuchterlein KH (1986). Symptom monitoring in the rehabilitation of schizophrenic patients. *Schizophrenia Bulletin*, **12**: 578–602.

McCrone P, Beecham J, Knapp MRJ (1994). Community psychiatric nurse teams: cost-effectiveness of intensive support versus generic care. *British Journal of Psychiatry*, **165**: 218–21.

Mangen SP, Paykel ES, Griffiths JH, Burchell A, Mancini P (1983). Cost-effectiveness of community psychiatric nurse or out-patient psychiatrist care of neurotic patients. *Psychological Medicine*, **13**: 407–16.

Marks IM, Connolly J, Muijen M, Audini B, McNamee G, Lawrence RE (1994). Home based versus hospital based care for people with serious mental illness: a controlled study. *British Journal of Psychiatry*, **165**: 179–94.

Maynard A (1993). Cost management: the economist's viewpoint. *British Journal of Psychiatry*, **163** (Suppl 20): 7–13.

Muijen M, Cooney M, Strathdee G, Bell R, Hudson A (1994). Community psychiatric nurse teams: intensive support versus generic care. *British Journal of Psychiatry*, **165**: 211–17 .

Netten A, Smart S (1993). *Unit Costs of Community Care*. PSSRU, Canterbury.
North C, Ritchie J (1993). *Factors Influencing the Implementation of the Care Programme Approach*. HMSO, London.
O'Donnell O (1991). Cost-effectiveness of community care for the chronic mentally ill. In: Freeman H, Henderson J (eds) *Evaluation of Comprehensive Care of the Mentally Ill*, Gaskell, London.
O'Driscoll C, Leff J (1993). The TAPS Project. 8: Design of the research study on the long-stay patients. *British Journal of Psychiatry*, **162** (Suppl. 19): 18–24.
Overall JE, Gorham DR (1962). Impact of treatment intervention on the relationship between dimensions of clinical psychopathology, social dysfunction and burden on the family of psychiatric patients. *British Journal of Psychiatry*, **12**: 651–8.
Schneider J (1993). Care programming in mental health: assimilation and adaptation. *British Journal of Social Work*, **23**: 383–403.
Schneider J (1995). Costing the care programme approach. In: Knapp MRJ (ed.) *The Economic Evaluation of Mental Health Services*, Ashgate, Aldershot.
Social Services Inspectorate (1992). *Community Care: Strategies for Implementation*. Department of Health, London.
Sturt E, Wykes T (1986). Assessment schedules for chronic psychiatric patients. *Psychological Medicine*, **17**: 485–93.
Sugden R, Williams A (1978). *The Principles of Practical Cost-Benefit Analysis*. Oxford University Press, Oxford.
Thomas CS, Stone K, Osborn M, Thomason PF, Fisher M (1993). Psychiatric morbidity and compulsory admission among UK-born Europeans, Afro-Caribbeans and Asians in central Manchester. *British Journal of Psychiatry*, **163**: 91–9.
Thornicroft G, Gooch C, O'Driscoll, Reda S (1993). The reliability of the patient attitude questionnaire. *British Journal of Psychiatry*, **162** (Suppl. 19): 25–9.
Weissman MM, Klerman GL, Paykel ES, Prusoff B, Hanson B (1974). Treatment effects on the social adjustment of depressed patients. *Archives of General Psychiatry*, **30**: 771–8.
Weissman MM, Paykel ES, Siegel R, Klerman G (1971). The social role performance of depressed women: comparisons with a normal group. *American Journal of Orthopsychiatry*, **41**: 390–405.
Wilkinson, G, Croft-Jerffreys C, Krekorian H, McLees S, Falloon I (1990). QALY's in psychiatric care? *Psychiatric Bulletin*, **14**: 582–5.
Wing JK, Cooper J, Sartorius N (1974). *The Measurement and Classification of Psychiatric Symptoms*. Cambridge University Press, Cambridge.
Wistow G, Knapp MRJ, Hardy B, Allen C (1994). *Social Care in a Mixed Economy*. Open University Press, Buckingham.

11

Future research strategies
Edited by PETER TYRER

Introduction

The last part of the meeting was devoted to a discussion about ideas for new research. The following chapter is an edited version of these contributions. The session was introduced by Professor Tom Craig who sought answers to two important questions that recurred frequently throughout the meeting; the choice of research design and the identification of the special ingredients that made for successful community care. The third issue that received considerable attention was that of training of staff in community psychiatry and the importance of research in evaluating this.

The randomised controlled trial

Many of the limitations of the randomised controlled trial were pointed out by the delegates. Such trials are ideal for comparing specific treatments, such as drugs, where a patient clearly receives one drug or the other. Service utilisation cannot be separated in the same way, although the methodology of the randomised controlled trial tends to force a Procrustean separation. Dr Burns felt that we were too preoccupied in separating hospital and non-hospital treatment. He argued that we were really comparing different ways of delivering services, both of which involved hospital treatment; in very few cases would no hospital treatment be used. The results of the studies described at the meeting (and abroad) showed that with good community care the degree of hospitalisation was reduced for a substantial number of patients. By reducing the overall need of most patients for hospital care important gains were achieved. This did not however mean that hospital care was inappropriate and it would be wrong to interpret the results in this way.

Dr Dean reinforced this argument by emphasising that we were comparing levels of care rather than hospital and community treatment. Sometimes patients needed intensive nursing care and at other times they did not. Efficient care meant having the intensive care available whenever the patients needed it. In a sophisticated service, such intensive care can be provided in the community.

Professor Marks argued that, despite their limitations, randomised controlled trials were still the best way of comparing therapeutic interventions and that we had not yet found a better methodology since Ronald Fisher made his pioneering agricultural studies in Rothamsted 70 years ago. Professor Murray suggested that there was 'a certain amount of self-congratulation' among the delegates because a set of consistent findings had been shown from randomised controlled studies. Many of these studies, however, were remarkably crude when compared, for example, with many drug trials. It was generally agreed among researchers in therapeutics that comparing unspecified interventions with unspecified patients in small numbers was quite inappropriate as a research strategy. It is necessary to specify in quite considerable detail whether improvement is in terms of diagnosis, symptoms or social functioning; which of the individuals were going to receive the intervention, its exact nature and the numbers needed for effective comparison. If this were possible we would be able to assess the value of a particular intervention in, for example, white, non-Afro-Caribbeans with schizophrenia rather than describing our population as those with 'severe mental illness', as is common at present.

Professor Murray was also concerned about the possible bias in findings introduced by the enthusiasts in many of these studies. In particular, the placebo effect seemed to be ignored. He knew of no studies in which a service run by enthusiasts was compared with one using similar methods but run by non-enthusiasts. There seemed little doubt that enthusiasm was an important ingredient of success but this was rarely controlled.

Professor Creed defended the randomised controlled studies that had already been carried out and discussed at the meeting. Certainly, the studies reported did not indicate which type of service was best for a specific patient but he queried whether the abundant literature on double-blind drug trials has informed us which antidepressant should be selected for a particular patient. He agreed that both those evaluating community psychiatry and those evaluating drug treatment needed to be able to define subgroups of patients, but both depended on large sample sizes, or similar trials that allow a meta-analysis. Such trials are difficult to fund in community psychiatry.

He did not exclude the possibility of combining the data from several studies on specific groups of patients (e.g. young male Afro-Caribbeans or others who were very high service users). Once it was possible to identify homogeneous subgroups within this population it might then be reasonable to carry out further studies (e.g. such as a drug trial of clozapine in high service users suffering from schizophrenia). He also queried the value of many of the lengthy instruments used in other randomised controlled trials such as the Present State Examination (PSE; Wing *et al.*, 1974). Much shorter assessments such as the Social Behaviour Schedule (SBS) (Sturt & Wykes, 1986) had been found to be very helpful in the hands of the Manchester group and Professor Creed suggested that many of the longer instruments could be substituted by short ones without loss of important information. This proposal was supported by Professor Tyrer, who commented that in his own work on services the assessments sometimes took considerably longer to complete than the treatments.

A great deal more information was needed about services in whole sectors or districts. The Nottingham data presented by Dr Ferguson were helpful and it was necessary to extend this to other areas. In collecting such data we needed more information about outcome. He mentioned a particular Director of Public Health in a district who had insisted, as part of his contract with the psychiatric services, that all patients who were admitted should have a PSE-like syndrome profile presented. This seems unnecessary and he preferred Dr Holloway's suggestion of addressing specific research questions with appropriate instruments for much smaller groups of patients.

Professor Murray responded by defending the use of instruments like the PSE in delineating the characteristics of subjects who might respond to particular interventions. A PSE profile would help, for example, in patients who are psychotic and who demonstrate mood disturbance. It has been shown that lithium may be more effective in such patients than a similar population which does not have mood disturbance and similarly if they have more typical psychotic symptoms then an antipsychotic drug may be more valuable (Johnstone *et al.*, 1988).

He thought it was important to identify subjects, for example with particular syndrome profiles, who were going to respond to psycho-social interventions or to a different form of management that would improve compliance with anti-psychotic drugs. Similarly, he asked whether individuals who become psychotic after experiencing major life events are more likely to respond to a type of community intervention which is going to diminish the likelihood of their suffering following further life events. He argued that now some of the basic studies have been done it was appropriate to move on to more precise questions.

As the final round in this interesting debate Professor Creed emphasised that there was a great deal of difference between deciding whether drug intervention was effective (e.g. lithium in bipolar affective psychosis) and deciding whether a patient needed admission to hospital. He commented that much of his own training suggested that certain syndromes necessitated hospital admission whereas his experience in community work had demonstrated that many of these could be treated successfully outside. This may explain the missionary zeal that sometimes accompanies discussions on community psychiatry.

Professor Marks added that the results of community care were not sufficient to justify any form of self-congratulation. He thought there was general agreement that community care did not cure serious mental illness; it made a small impact and it did lead to greater patient satisfaction and was marginally less expensive than inpatient based care. What he found impressive was the similarity of these findings across different studies, whether they were carried out in London, Sydney or Wisconsin. In this respect, a consensus was beginning to develop which was as impressive as that for lithium in mood disorders. (Although he thought all of us needed to be modest, he did not think it necessary to be any more modest than our colleagues in other areas.)

From a scientific methodological standpoint Dr Lewis asked the delegates to look objectively at the studies that had been presented during the course of this symposium. He noted that all the studies had a relatively small sample size, despite the hard work that had gone into collecting the data. He also noted that no one had given confidence intervals for the size of the effects being found (although these are presented in some of the published data) and he wondered how many other important effects were hidden away in the data that were being presented. Naturally, much of the focus of research was on clinical and social outcome. As an objective observer, he felt that any benefits for community care appeared to be fairly marginal and it would not be appropriate to change national policy on the basis of a few significant results here and there that showed benefit for community treatment. If, however, there were sufficient numbers in the studies, it might be possible to demonstrate a definite advantage of one treatment over another. This would be a more robust finding and it is quite possible that it would be more valuable than the relatively gross differences that have been detected in the individual studies to date.

He also queried whether we were measuring the right outcomes. We concentrate on the organisation of care but the outcomes were usually examining only clinical and social outcome. Clearly, costs were important and it was relevant that in almost all the studies presented a consistent finding was that it was much cheaper to treat people in the community, although this might not be true for the most severely dependent people. The outcome in terms of staff attitudes and morale was equally important.

Dr Lewis also made the important point that the randomised controlled trial would become increasingly difficult to operate because there are few areas left in which parallel services exist. In a district such as Sparkbrook in Birmingham, where Dr Dean's service was situated, it was clear that the area received a total package of care and that it was extremely difficult to imagine randomisation of patients in such a service. He thought the point was near when randomised studies, particularly those concerned with the organisation of services, might not be feasible research options.

Alternatives to randomised controlled trials

Dr Wykes expressed concern that so little attention had been paid to the functioning of staff in community teams in any of the studies presented during the symposium. She asked for evidence that posts in the community were attractive to professionals and could be sustained. Moving out into the community affects all psychiatric workers, in particular the effects on promotion prospects which, if poor, would make these jobs unattractive to all psychiatric professionals. Although these are not specific research projects they are extremely important in clinical practice. She asked what basic information was available on staff turnover in community teams and whether information was available on untoward instances to professionals in community teams? This information will be needed when organising training programmes.

We also needed more information for future research about basic questions on service organisation such as housing provision. For example, was it better to have one big hostel with 20 people rather than four hostels with five people in each. The single house will be cheaper and the outcome may well be the same. However, it is likely that the users would say that they would rather have the smaller houses.

There could be very negative effects, however, which Dr Wykes referred to as toxic ones (an adjective that was taken up by other delegates during the course of the discussion) which had yet to be identified. Is living with staff in a large hostel toxic? What factors in a psychiatric patient's environment might make community care fail? The building evaluation unit of the Department of Health (DoH) which if it still exists might be able to advise on the design of mental health buildings for community provision.

Dr Wykes suggested capitalising on smaller studies and data from natural experiments which would be extremely valuable in specifying factors predictive of good and poor outcomes. She cited the natural experiment going on at the Maudsley Hospital at the current time in which each sector was producing a different model of service which would allow comparison between sectors. This information alone, however, would not be of value because everyone regarded the Maudsley Hospital as atypical, so it was necessary to get details from other natural experiments going on elsewhere. The randomised controlled trial could only compare a few key variables; natural experiments such as this could look at many more.

Professor Knapp followed on from this by describing his examination of 28 projects around England which were funded by the DoH under the care and community demonstration programme. These covered a range of different groups; there were seven or eight for mental health problems, 12 for learning disabilities and so on. They all sought to move long-stay patients into the community but set up different models of care.

Professor Knapp's team evaluated all 28 using the same instrumentation and therefore had a natural experiment already set up. They found for example that staff working in small group homes, unstaffed group homes, peripatetic staff and those involved in adult fostering arrangements had high burdens imposed on them and this led to a high turnover of staff. They also found that in the group who had learning difficulties the characteristics of the care environment and the settings in which people lived were very important predictors of outcome. He felt that the data presented at the symposium had not been sufficiently analysed and that further scrutiny might help to understand which people do particularly well in one service and badly in another. It would be very difficult to incorporate these into a randomised controlled design at this stage because several factors were involved but we should not be too restrictive. It was often possible to extrapolate from one study to another and postulate that the indicators of good progress in one group could be incorporated into another study. In his conversations with statisticians these suggestions normally met with horror but he felt they should be taken more seriously.

Dr Melzer suggested that there was a false antithesis between the randomised controlled trial and survey and observation techniques. He felt there were two necessary elements. The first was to define whether specific interventions are effective and this could only be satisfactorily answered using the randomised controlled trial. The second is to find out whether, in practice, the service delivered to ordinary people in the NHS through a variety of different providers, including social services, fundholders, the benefit system and the psychiatric services, was functioning well. He felt that there was too much unnecessary confusion between these separate elements. There was a need for both descriptive studies and formative evaluations: evaluations aimed at getting us a better service using techniques that we know are effective. We do not need a trial for these elements.

Professor Marks commented on Dr Lewis' observation that the sample sizes were too small in many of the investigations. Even in the 189 cases identified in the Daily Living Project (DLP) there were insufficient numbers to identify subgroups. The standard method of improving the sample was to do multi-site studies. Examples of these include the National Institutes of Mental Health (NIMH) depression study in which antidepressants, cognitive and interpersonal therapy were compared (Elkin *et al.*, 1989). These studies were expensive but there is no reason why several funding bodies should not combine to support these important studies. It was only by getting large enough numbers that we could start asking questions about the various subgroups of patients that were necessary in planning services.

He also agreed that it was extremely important to find out whether treatment methods and approaches were sustainable. Unfortunately, the measures that were generally used in research designs were much too cumbersome to be used in routine practice. If we wanted to ensure that the standard of care was being maintained, then it was reasonable to ask trainees to apply some simple, well-tried measure of outcome in their patients to show that they were achieving the effects for which they had been trained. To do this we badly needed some simpler measures of outcome and also simple summaries of the skills that were being employed but it should not be too difficult to evolve these. If it became a normal expectation that workers in the field should use these simple measures to track both their work and the outcome of the patients then we would have made a great step forward.

Professor Tyrer commented on Dr Strathdee's suggestion that natural experiments currently being introduced into the health service should be evaluated. He said that this was a unique time in the health service in which a great deal of change was going on to evaluate as many of these changes as possible, possibly with the help of organisations such as Research and Development for Psychiatry (RDP) and others, who could use the same evaluations in all cases.

Identification of subgroups for study

Dr Muijen maintained that we should move on to study different types of aftercare in the community. It is being shown clearly that community care with intensive aftercare was highly superior when compared with hospital admission followed by virtually no aftercare and it was unnecessary to repeat these studies. It was extremely important, however, to know what 'density of care' was needed for which subgroups and how the service should be delivered. Professor Marks commented on recent work involved with families of schizophrenics which showed positive findings. As only about 25% of the schizophrenic patients included in the studies were discussed at the symposium, these findings could not be generalisable to all psychotic patients.

Professor Creed repeated the question that Dr Holloway had made in his presentation, which is almost a universal one in psychiatry, which patients need which treatment? Professor Creed thought that because of his training, the appropriate split was a diagnostic one but in recent months he had wondered whether it should be defined by severity of illness. He pointed to the example of some severely ill patients who do not have schizophrenia but nonetheless, as Martin Knapp had pointed out, have high service use and it may be possible to categorise patients in this way alone. He thought that high service use and severity of illness might be more highly correlated with the need for community care than diagnostic labels.

The organisation of care was important in an intervention such as the family treatment of schizophrenia. For example, recruitment might be affected by whether the patient was first assessed at home or in hospital or at the beginning or end of an acute illness. In the day hospital or community setting staff, patient and carers have to work much more closely than they ever do with inpatient treatment. This might help to establish a kind of therapeutic rapport between staff and relatives which will enable a far greater proportion of relatives to engage in family treatment than is currently the case. This could be tested in a study which assessed recruitment and outcome of family therapy for patients with schizophrenia in the ward and in the day hospital.

Dr Wykes thought it was useful looking at diagnostic groups. If, for example, we believe that young male manic patients require hospitalisation this is something we could test with our current data. What will be much more informative for services and future research however, is to identify the toxic effects in service delivery. Who were the people who could not be contained in a community environment and what were the reasons behind their admission? Was it their level of symptomatology or was it because they were a danger to themselves and others? There should be factors which we could define on the basis of our current patient population.

Barbara Tomenson commented that Professor Knapp's data seemed to suggest that inpatient care was better for a small number of patients but community care was better for a much larger number. What was needed was how best to assign the patients to the different arms of the service. Was this a reasonable way of choosing the type of service? Would, for example, young male schizophrenic Afro-Caribbeans be best treated as inpatients and others in the community?

Training of staff for community care

Dr Melzer asked what would be the ideal composition of a multi-disciplinary community psychiatric team. In the formal presentations there was a fairly standard description of team members but little discussion about the exact qualities and qualifications of each team member. For example, there was a lot of discussion in community teams about the role of the care assistant. How much can care assistants be used in this type of treatment? Professor Tyrer referred to the blurring of roles in a community team. If there really were so much blurring of roles why do we have such wage differentials between different workers? Have any of the studies examined these issues?

Richard Ford responded by saying that case managers who were non-qualified seemed to stay only a short time in their posts although there had been no formal comparisons of the clients for whom care assistants were responsible compared with those clients of those carers who had a professional qualification.

Professor Marks said he was surprised when designing the DLP study in 1987 that there was no training programme for community care worthy of the name. The Australian and Madison studies could only pass on details of their training by discussion and this was a major problem in setting up the DLP. The initial training programme was 'boot-strapped' but became more comprehensive over time. There were now programmes for training on expressed emotion in schizophrenia, the problem centred approach that had been adopted from Madison and behavioural psychological treatment. These could now all be combined in a single package of training. We could not maintain that this was the optimum package as there may be other aspects such as suicide prevention which are equally important.

Professor Tyrer thought that Professor Marks' suggestion was an excellent one and that, with his previous experience, he would be an excellent person to get it off the ground. Another aspect of this issue was that reaching people who needed the help of the community team was at least as important as the nature of the treatment given and this depended a lot on the quality and training of staff in community teams. In the Early Intervention Service (EIS) in Paddington, and with Dr Burns' service at St George's, it had been found that one of the main advantages of the community care approach was that many more people were engaged than in the standard type of service (Merson *et al.*, 1992). User satisfaction was clearly not the same as outcome but it was still extremely important as patients who preferred being seen in the community and liked this approach were more likely to respond to the therapeutic measures given because they were would be more compliant. Getting people to want to see you requires a certain sort of training in itself and this could be included in a package as well as the formal training skills. This issue has tended to be disregarded in traditional practice because much hospital work involves captive populations.

Gary McNamee reinforced the need for research into the training of nurses in particular as they were still the largest element of the community care workforce. It was important to know whether we could attract good people for this task. The training course to which Professor Marks had referred was about to enter its first real year of operation. Even before the notice of such training became publicly available, subscription rates to it by nurses throughout the country became quite overwhelming. This seems to indicate that even those already working in the field feel they desperately need additional help. This request from the grass roots for support, training and skills appears to be evidence of the need to have such training, following which we would need to research the consequences of the training process in terms of outcome.

Dr Burns commented that, in his experience, it was nurses who expanded their role most greatly when they were attached to community teams. Their experience of working outside the hospital in a slightly different setting liberated them and allowed them to use a whole range of skills (for which they may not have been fully trained) which were quite different skills from their previous work. He thought it was important that the dormant skills, which had never had the opportunity to fully develop, should be identified in selecting people for this type of work. One of the most obvious ones was commonsense. He was surprised that this was frequently only apparent outside hospital because it was only in these settings that workers had a much wider range of choice and scope. It might be of interest to see the value of training exercises in order to examine what people do when they are given different options and allowed the opportunity to work in a different way.

Gary McNamee commented that one of the reasons why people were keen on joining community services was that the pressures facing staff in the acute hospital services were so great that it was understandable that they were leaving in large numbers. This did not mean that we would necessarily hold on to staff in community care unless we were able to give them something better. He emphasised the need for research to develop the necessary skills both in enhancing outcomes of care and in giving satisfaction to staff so that they remained within the service.

Professor Creed thought that it was imperative in future studies to look at data about staff turnover, staff morale and other elements of staff satisfaction. There was no reason why data already collected should not be combined to see exactly what were the specific features that lead to a high staff turnover so that these could be avoided in the future. Specific studies were needed on these issues, not just as by-products of other work. Professor Tyrer stressed that one of the major problems in getting community teams to work together in a truly multi-disciplinary way was the absence of a common training programme for staff in community care. What was needed is a qualification for community psychiatric practice which was available across disciplines. This would be difficult to develop because of the territorial nature of different disciplines within the psychiatric professions but the need for such a qualification was still there. Working across disciplines was difficult but was made unnecessarily more difficult because of our variation in training. Once there was a common qualification for community staff the functioning of multi-disciplinary teams would become much easier.

Future directions

Dr Wykes came back to the need to have simple measures of outcome to make it easier for all community team members to record progress of care. She thought that it would be quite unnecessary to use instruments such as the PSE because they were never really envisaged as measures of change. There had been other studies with instruments such as the SBS (Sturt & Wykes, 1986) but there was a need for other instruments that could be used in many countries to allow comparison of data.

Professor Marks said that one of the most important items of measurement was the economic analysis. Unfortunately, this involved collecting a lot of data and it was difficult to see how this could be streamlined. Professor Knapp responded that because the various forms of overnight accommodation such as inpatient care and imprisonment, together with day hospital activity, were the most expensive items of care a streamlined list such as this one was extremely valuable. Dr Kingdon responded on behalf of the DoH to many of the points that had been raised. He referred back to 1975 and the publication of *Better Services for the Mentally Ill* (HMSO, 1975) and specifically to compare the aspirations in that document with the situation that existed now. He maintained that what was written in *Better Services for the Mentally Ill* was not very different from present policy and that the achievements since 1975 had confirmed that the aims of that White Paper were the correct ones. The findings of the studies presented at the symposium had, in effect, confirmed the approach set out in the 1975 document as the correct one and therefore may have relatively little effect on influencing current policy. He felt that where research was particularly important is in persuading colleagues in the psychiatric professions to implement the ideas that have now been in circulation for a long time. What was it that at present stops them from being disseminated and implemented?

He thought that the blame could not be laid at the purchasers' door. Although many of the initiatives had been led professionally (individuals such as Tom Burns had initiated and developed a service because it seemed to be the right way forward) but resources had subsequently been available to fund this. Although some teams had been set up specifically for research many of the presentations at the symposium had been, in effect, on the back of existing teams and services. It was the attitudes that were the key to successful implementation. He thought that we needed further research into attitudes; specifically, the methods of changing our colleagues' attitudes who seemed to be blind to these developments.

He agreed that there was a high priority in establishing good measures of outcome. This was currently being addressed by the research team at the Royal College of Psychiatrists under Professor Wing. He was not sure whether this was going to produce a research instrument or, more likely, a practical outcome measure that could be used at local level for people to audit their own services. It may be that there are particular elements of these measures that we ought to be using regularly rather than having the comprehensive range that we have at present. Perhaps only one or two measures from the PSE were useful with the groups that we were studying and the same may well apply to the Social Behaviour Assessment Schedule (SBAS; Platt *et al.*, 1980) and similar instruments.

He agreed that it was likely that there was much in the existing data that had not been presented at the symposium that could be very valuable in giving ideas for future studies. If we thought of the work described at this meeting as pilot studies there appeared to be common trends that could be used in new projects. There was a particular need to identify, from the hierarchy of interventions that services could be using, which were the most successful and should be used most frequently.

Judy Harrison commented from the viewpoint of someone who had been both a psychiatric provider and a public health doctor. Her view was that most purchasers were ahead of us in wanting to move faster towards community care. She did not think that purchasers were holding us back at all; it was the providers who were reluctant to consider community care for a number of reasons. She thought that there was a fear of change for people who were already quite burnt-out in providing a service and that perhaps we had concentrated too much at the meeting on the research aspect of our work and not enough on the development one. It was necessary to find out ways of encouraging our colleagues who worked in community services to take on the care of those patients that would radically reduce the rate of hospital admissions and the need for hospital based services. We need to look in more detail at what these interventions are and for which patients they are most suitable. We may have shown that it is possible to reduce bed usage quite markedly but our purchasers are really ahead of us in asking for more information to enhance these figures. Clearly our intervention may prevent admission but if admission would not be necessary in any case this would not be valuable.

Professor Craig terminated the meeting by summarising the need to identify both the positive and toxic effects of our interventions more accurately and to support the notion of setting up a large multi-centre study that could look at sufficiently large numbers of patients to answer many of the questions that had been posed by the delegates during the meeting. He also commented on the universal enthusiasm for training community staff, particularly nurses, and the potential value of the Thorn nurse training programme which was just about to be implemented. The discussion had emphasised that a radically different approach was necessary for those working in the community and we now had sufficient information about the type of skills needed to offer an adequate training programme. As a final comment he reiterated the need for a quick and easy measure for recording outcomes rather than those which were laborious and of high intensity.

References

Elkin I, Shea MT, Watkins JT *et al.* (1989). National Institute of Mental health treatment of depression collaborative research program: general effectiveness of treatments. *Archives of General Psychiatry*, **46**: 971–82.

HMSO (1975). *Better Services for the Mentally Ill*. HMSO, London.

Johnstone EC, Crow TJ, Frith CD, Owens DGC (1988). The Northwick Park 'Functional' Psychosis Study: diagnosis and treatment response. *Lancet*, **ii**: 119–26.

Merson S, Tyrer P, Onyett S *et al.* (1992). Early intervention in psychiatric emergencies: a controlled clinical trial. *Lancet*, **339**: 1311–14.

Platt S, Weyman A, Hirsch S, Hewett S (1980). The Social Behaviour Assessment Schedule (SBAS): rationale, contents, scoring and reliability of a new interview schedule. *Social Psychiatry*, **15**: 43–55.

Sturt E, Wykes T (1986). The Social Behaviour Schedule: a validity and reliability study. *British Journal of Psychiatry*, **148**: 1–11.

Wing JK, Cooper JE, Sartorius N (1974). *The Measurement and Classification of Psychiatric Symptoms*. Cambridge University Press, Cambridge.

Index